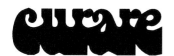

ZEITSCHRIFT FÜR MEDIZINETHNOLOGIE
JOURNAL OF MEDICAL ANTHROPOLOGY

hg. von der Arbeitsgemeinschaft Ethnologie und Medizin (AGEM)
ed. by the Association for Anthropology and Medicine (AGEM)

VOL. 45 (2022) 2

Editorial

Wann beginnt menschliches Leben und wann endet es? Lebensanfänge und -enden sind intensive, aber auch intensiv diskutierte Momente, die weit über intime Situationen hinausgehen. Bioethische Gesetze zu ungeborenem Leben, Debatten zu Hirntod und Sterbehilfe oder weltweite Rückschritte in reproduktiven Rechten sind nur vier von vielen Themen, in denen die Grenzen von Leben, Lebensfähigkeit, Recht auf Leben und gutem Leben politisch und sozial verhandelt werden. Der vorliegende Schwerpunkt mit dem Titel „Ethnographische Erkundungen und methodologische Reflexionen über Lebensanfänge und -enden" zeigt sensibel auf, wie ethische und methodologische Herausforderungen, die sich bei Forschungen an Lebensanfängen und -enden stellen, ein Prisma für ethnographisches Arbeiten allgemein sind. Die Herausgeberinnen JULIA REHSMANN & VERONIKA SIEGL lassen klassische und neuere medizinanthropologische Auseinandersetzungen mit Lebensanfängen und -enden Revue passieren, und demonstrieren, welche Politiken des Lebens und Sterbens dabei auf dem Spiel stehen. In den drei Forschungsartikeln, die Rehsmann und Siegl für den Schwerpunkt versammelt haben, wird deutlich, dass Fragen von Feldzugang, Positionalität, Verantwortung und Forschungsethik eine besondere Aufmerksamkeit zuteil wird, die in weniger sensiblen ethnographischen Forschungsfeldern bisweilen zu sehr in den Hintergrund rücken.

In einem von dem Schwerpunkt unabhängigen Artikel widmet sich der Arzt und Religionswissenschaftler JÜRGEN W. DOLLMANN der Frage nach der Verwendung des Begriffs der Ganzheitlichkeit in Komplementär- und Alternativmedizin. Im Anschluss führen wir unsere mittlerweile etablierte Rubrik „Lehrforum" fort, in der diesmal zum einen LISA LEHNER & MAGDALENA EITENBERGER über das multimediale Arbeiten und das Verhältnis von Wissenschaft und Öffentlichkeit nachdenken und zum anderen MARÍA FERNANDA OLARTE-SIERRA über *care* und Verletzlichkeit beim Unterrichten der Themen Tod und Verlust reflektiert.

Nachdem wir mit dem vergangenen Heft zum Reimer-Verlag gewechselt sind, kommt ab dem kommenden Jahr eine weitere Neuerung hinzu, denn ab 2023 wird die *Curare* als Open Access Zeitschrift erscheinen, wobei wir weiterhin eine Druckversion bereitstellen werden.

Zuletzt möchten wir noch auf die nächste Jahrestagung der AGEM hinweisen, die unter dem Titel „Krisen, Körper, Kompetenzen: Methoden und Potentiale medizinanthropologischen Forschens" in Kooperation mit der Kommission Medizinanthropologie der Deutschen Gesellschaft für Empirische Kulturwissenschaft (DGEKW) vom 8.–9. September 2023 im Warburg Haus in Hamburg stattfinden wird. Ein Call for Papers findet sich am Ende dieser Ausgabe.

DIE REDAKTION

SCHWERPUNKT
THEMATIC FOCUS

Beginnings and Ends of Life
Ethnographic Explorations and Methodological Reflections

EDITED BY
JULIA REHSMANN & VERONIKA SIEGL

The Beginnings and Ends of Life as a Magnifying Glass for Ethnographic Research

Introduction to the Special Issue

JULIA REHSMANN & VERONIKA SIEGL

With bans on assisted suicide recently ended in several European states, such as Germany and Austria, and (quasi) bans on abortion recently reinstated in Poland and the United States but lifted in countries such as Ireland, Colombia and Argentina, public discourse around the boundaries of life and death, and whose right it is to decide for or against them, has become highly politicized. The recent political developments prove that it is no longer possible to take once-established rights and restrictions for granted. A critical engagement with the beginnings and ends of life is thus timely, for scholars and activists alike.

Being universal and fundamentally life-changing human experiences (WOJTKOWIAK & MATHIJSSEN 2022), the beginnings and ends of life can serve as a productive prism through which to understand society and culture (AULINO 2019; DAVIS-FLOYD 2019; GARCIA 2016; GINSBURG & RAPP 1995; KAUFMAN 2015; LOCK 2002; VAN HOLLEN 2003). Taking this as a starting point, we argue that these experiences also serve as a magnifying glass for issues inherent in anthropological research and ethnographic fieldwork, while posing new questions relevant to an academic field that is called upon to remain self-critical and re-evaluate long-held traditions and taken-for-granted research practices, such as pseudonymization or conducting participant observation in sensitive contexts.

These questions are the focus of the present special issue, which brings together ethnographic research on the beginnings and ends of life, from MARCOS ANDRADE NEVES on transnational assisted suicide across Germany, the UK and Switzerland, to MIRA MENZFELD on dying in Germany and MOLLY FITZPATRICK on "natural birth" in Indonesia. This introduction will provide a conceptual and empirical framework for the three contributions. In the first part, we

briefly sketch how the beginnings and ends of life have been researched within anthropology, argue for the productivity of bringing these seemingly oppositional phenomena together and raise questions about the particularities of ethnographic research at the beginnings and ends of life. In the second part, we turn our attention to the politics of life and death. We show that, while the beginnings and ends of life are universal experiences, the way these play out in individual people's lives is highly structured by intersecting inequalities. In the concluding section, we return to the methodological issues raised above and introduce the individual contributions in greater detail.

Bringing the Beginnings and Ends of Life Together

Ethnographic engagements with the beginnings and ends of life have a long history within social anthropology. As SHARON KAUFMAN and LYNN MORGAN (2005) show in their elaborate review essay, this engagement has been subject to major transformations over time. While earlier studies scrutinized the beginnings and ends of life through the prism of structural-functionalism and in relation to religion, ritual, kinship and social cohesion, more recent studies have addressed these phenomena through the lenses of political economy, poststructuralism, globalization and postcolonialism (KAUFMAN & MORGAN 2005: 318f). They have shed light on local accommodations and adaptations of globally circulating bioscience, technologies, ethics and biopolitics, and expanded understandings of the affects, materialities and involvement of non-human actors at the beginnings and ends of life. Moreover, research in and beyond anthropology has pointed to the ambiguous boundaries between life and death – revealing how these are shaped by cultural, political and scientific negotiations (BENKEL & MEITZLER 2021; DAS & HAN 2016; KAUFMAN & MORGAN 2005, NIEDER & SCHNEIDER 2007) and pointing to the many ways in which life and death, care and violence, illness and healing fold into each other. The beginnings and ends of life, thus, cover a multitude of very different biological processes, social events and subjective experiences, including various forms birth, assisted reproduction, embryonic stem cell research, abortion, pre- and perinatal death, organ transplants, palliative care, assisted suicide, euthanasia, cryonics or spiritual ideas around afterlife and reincarnation.

Reflecting on the connections between the beginnings and ends of life offers productive opportunities for anthropologists to unpack methodological concerns that become highlighted by the particularities of these existential, and liminal, phenomena – an issue that so far little has been written about. It was exactly this reflection that formed the starting point for the present special issue. Our own research on commercial surrogacy and selective abortion (SIEGL 2018a, 2018b, forthcoming 2023) as well as organ transplants and palliative care (REHSMANN 2018, 2021, 2022; SOOM AMMANN & REHSMANN 2022) had spurred countless conversations between us and made us realize that we were grappling with similar methodological puzzles in very different research settings. Both being interested in the role of affects and emotions in ethnographic fieldwork (REHSMANN 2019; SIEGL 2019), we wanted to investigate the obstacles and opportunities that ethnographic explorations in these existential settings present for us as researchers, and how they complicate long-held anthropological assumptions concerning participant observation, as well as notions like vulnerability, emotionality and intimacy. Our interest in these questions was also fuelled by the way friends, relatives or fellow researchers reacted to the topics of our research – often with awe, commenting on how they thought these topics must be "depressing" or somehow particularly "difficult" to work on. But why are these topics thought to be more challenging than others?

Discussing the end of life, MARIAN KRAWCZYK and NAOMI RICHARDS (2021: 409) criticize assumptions that ethnographic research in this field poses more emotional challenges and requires more emotional intimacy than other fields of study. The authors argue against a romanticized view of ethnographic research on dying, that is, against an othering of this existential experience as inherently apart from other aspects of everyday life. While we fully support this argument, we contend that research on birthing and dying cannot be fully equated with other everyday experiences. Even following an integrative approach towards dying as part of life, questions to us as anthropologists nonetheless remain: What *are* the particularities of conducting research at the beginnings and ends of life? Are these settings somehow more intimate than others, do they require other modes of 'being-with', witnessing and participating? Are the research participants we encounter at the beginnings and ends of life somehow more vulnerable than others? How do we make sense of the existential gap between research participants and anthropologists conducting fieldwork on these matters? The "strength of the anthropological approach", as SJAAK VAN DER GEEST (2007: 10) puts it, lies in its transparency regarding its limits in fully capturing experiences of "pain, illness and suffering". If we accept the need for transparent humility, critical attentiveness and emotional reflexivity, ethnographic research on the beginnings and ends of life calls on us to look closely into the particularities of these settings, asking how they play out in anthropological research and what they tell us about the fields themselves.

The Politics of Life and Death

The fact that all human beings are born and die is often used as a basis to argue that we are all equal in relation to these existential events. Likewise, early anthropological engagements with these topics were often merely descriptive and comparative, focusing on how the beginnings and ends of life were shaped in specific cultures (e. g. HERTZ 1960; JORDAN 1978). Regarding the beginnings of life, it was only with the influence of the feminist movements in the 1970s and 1980s that scholarly engagement gradually became more analytical and political, with classic works by, for example, FAYE D. GINSBURG and RAYNA RAPP

(1995) or ROBBIE DAVIS-FLOYD (1992). Such later engagements have shown that birth and death are not uniform processes but rather are determined by factors such as race, class, gender, dis/ability, religion, nationality and others, as well as being entangled in local and global relations of power (DAS & HAN 2016; ENGELKE 2019; GINSBURG & RAPP 1995). Life and death, as these later works highlight, are inherently political.

The recently published report of the Lancet Commission on the Value of Death, for instance, refers to dying in the 21st century as a "story of paradox" (SALLNOW ET AL. 2022: 837) and stresses the global imbalance of some people being overtreated in hospitals, while most people worldwide remain un- or undertreated, lack sufficient access to healthcare or are even left to die. These unequal and deadly dynamics are captured by ACHILLE MBEMBE's (2003) concept of "necropolitics" and are also analyzed ethnographically in the works of JOÃO BIEHL (2001) and NANCY SCHEPER-HUGHES (1993), both of whom tease out the connections between poverty, marginalization, neglect and death in Brazil. Linking the beginnings and ends of life, recent works have revealed the immense impact of race and racialization on pregnancy, labour and maternal death in the United States (DAVIS 2019; MULLINGS 2021) or the impact of a highly bureaucratic postcolonial health system on maternal death in rural Tanzania (STRONG 2020). Here, the concept of "stratified reproduction" (COLEN 1995; GINSBURG & RAPP 1995) has been productive in order to think through the ways in which the reproductive futures of some are encouraged, while those of others are inhibited – be it through high rates of maternal mortality, through forced or state-encouraged sterilization of peasant and working-class women (CHAPARRO-BUITRAGO 2022; RUDRAPPA 2012) or through the unequal distribution of and access to assisted and selective reproductive technologies (GAMMELTOFT &WAHLBERG 2014; INHORN 2021; NAHMAN 2016). Reproductive futures are also at stake in relation to the perceived safety of IVF treatments and the scientific and societal ignorance of the potentially harmful long-term effects of hormonal treatments, and the politico-economic dimensions that underlie these entanglements (JAIN 2013).

The development and spread of assisted reproductive technologies across the globe, particularly in high-income countries and among those with the means to afford them, are exemplary of the global rise of biomedicine. This rise has led to an increasing biomedicalization of birth and death with its focus on, among other things, epi/genetic risks, new diagnostic procedures and technoscientific innovations (CLARKE ET AL. 2003; CLARKE & SHIM 2011; DAVIS-FLOYD 1992; JORDAN 1993; KAUFMAN 2005, 2015; MARTIN 2001), with significant consequences for how birthing and dying are understood and practised. Under this "medical gaze" (FOUCAULT 2003), birthing and dying have moved from the home, family and community to clinical spaces – their "management", thus, increasingly learned in institutions (Davenport 2000) and shut out of everyday life and familiar spaces (FRASER 1995; GOTTLIEB 1995; VAN HOLLEN 2003). This move came along with the devaluation of traditional knowledge and of the expertise of female-dominated fields like nursing and midwifery, being replaced by the authority of mostly *white*,[1] male biomedical knowledge. This knowledge constructed the reproductive and the dying body as risky and flawed, in need of intervention, management and correction (CHADWICK & FOSTER 2014; DAVIS-FLOYD 1994; KAUFMAN 2015; MARTIN 2001; ROSE 2007; SIEGL 2018a). Counterintuitively, the move to the clinic has also cast the beginnings and ends of life as moments of ultimate privacy and vulnerability – moments that, thus, need to remain hidden in patients' rooms and well-guarded by clinical gatekeepers. This has had a fundamental impact on the im/possibilities of ethnographic research in such settings. While the introduction of ethics committees and informed consent procedures is, surely, to be welcomed in the context of clinic research, the streamlined approval forms, questionnaires and study protocols often fail to acknowledge the qualitative nature of anthropological research – with its explorative and relational approach, its focus on open and narrative interviews as well as its inherently situative ethics. Furthermore, questions of pseudonymization, anonymization, of un/naming research participants, organizations and institutions are very differently framed and negotiated from a clinical or an anthropological ethics perspective. The move to the clinic has, thus, rendered much ethnographic research on the beginnings and ends of life difficult and almost impossible to conduct. Our own experiences in this field suggest that talk about "privacy" and "vulnerability", while primarily brought forward in the name of patients' interests, also serves to ward off critical research altogether (SIEGL forthcoming 2023). As a consequence, many supposedly ethical questions are increasingly turned into political ones, determined by the interests of individual clinics with their entanglements with pharma and other industries.

The move to the clinic and, with it, the increasing biomedicalization (CLARKE ET AL. 2003) and technologization around reproduction and end-of-life care have allowed lives to be extended or ended, dying to be postponed or hastened, births to be scheduled, "anormal" pregnancies to be terminated, or reproduction to be outsourced or put on hold. These developments have significantly contributed to the re/making of life and death (ADRIAN 2020). As KAUFMAN and MORGAN point out, for those with access to the "new biomedical techniques, one's corporal materiality no longer imposes strict limits on the body or self" (2005: 330). This renegotiation of what were previously considered the natural limits of human life is tightly linked to the notions of (individual) choice and self-responsibility (RAPP 1999; ROSE 2007). Choices are never neutral but carry a moral imperative; it is the "right" or "appropriate" choice one must make, carrying with it the ever-dooming risk of choosing "wrongly". Recent ethnographies have shown the many ways in which people's dying and end-of-life are "choreographed" (STONINGTON 2020) and "scripted" (BUCHBINDER 2021), and how end-of-life decision-making is tied up with cultural complexities that question Western understandings of the individual and their rational decision-making (STAVRIANAKIS 2019; ZIVKOVIC 2021). Choices in the context of the beginnings and ends of life are saturated with ideas of potential and risks, of what these could be, of that which might happen. Choices around prenatal tests, choices about implantation, choices for or against life-prolonging treatments, choosing to end a life – one's own or that of another. Weighing risks, uncertainties and the *potential* consequences of one's choices. While

the contributions in this special issue focus on research outside the classical clinical institutions, they all relate to them, and partly come into being by people's choices to look for an alternative to biomedical approaches and clinical settings, from the choice to have a 'natural birth' in midwifery clinics (FITZPATRICK 2022), to deciding to end one's life in the flat of an assisted suicide organization (ANDRADE NEVES 2022), to the choices of terminally ill people in private homes and hospices (MENZFELD 2022). And yet: for most of the world's population, choices remain limited by unequal access to healthcare and it is those with more resources who are given the option to choose – be it the choice between clinics, for or against clinics, or for more or less medical intervention or care.

Methodological Reflections on Studying the Beginnings and Ends of Life

Reflections on the unequal dimensions of life and death are relevant not just in relation to the research topic per se but also in relation to methodological questions – including our positionality as anthropologists, own involvement in the fields we study and the entanglements between our private and professional lives.

Many scholars have detailed how ethnographic knowledge informs their personal encounters with the beginnings and ends of life, and vice versa – whether in the context of birth (GOTTLIEB 1995), assisted reproduction (JAIN 2013), pre- and perinatal loss (ADRIAN 2020; LAYNE 2003), the loss of friends and relatives (BEHAR 1996; REHSMANN 2019; ROSALDO 1993; WACKERS 2016) as well as own experiences with life-threatening diagnoses (JAIN 2013; MARKS 2012). These accounts show how personal encounters can offer a "cognitive opening" (DAS 2020: 316) to understanding such existential experiences. Of these personal accounts, RUTH BEHAR's book *The Vulnerable Observer* (1996) is probably one of the most cherished ones, arguing that we should not try to separate the person from the anthropologist, but we need to make visible and work with our own histories, experiences and emotions. With this argument, BEHAR echoes other feminist calls for acknowledging the positionality, intersectionality and shifting power relations in fieldwork settings

(ABU-LUGHOD 1990; BEHAR & GORDON 1995; DA-VIS & CRAVEN 2016; HARAWAY 1988; HARDING 2004; OAKLEY 1981; STACEY 1988).

What heightens the importance of reflecting on these issues in fieldwork settings at the beginnings and ends of life is the fact that both research participants and researcher often enter these settings without knowing beforehand how to negotiate them. Giving birth, at least for the first time, is not an "ordinary" experience in a person's life, as is dying. With little or no experience to draw upon, these encounters involve a lot of uncertainty. This aspect is taken up by MIRA MENZFELD'S contribution to this special issue. Drawing on Turner's thoughts on threshold and transition dynamics, MENZFELD argues that her ethnographic fieldwork with dying people in Germany was often marked by what she calls "liminal asymmetries" – since she herself was neither confronted with a lethal diagnosis nor in the process of dying herself. "Liminal asymmetries" refers to the fact that the dying find themselves in a betwixt-and-between state, from which they wish for a kind of liminal guidance and companionship that the researcher herself cannot offer; as well as the fact that there are crucial experience hierarchies in these research relationships, since the dying inhabit a very different mode of being and regard themselves as less privileged and agentic than the researcher. MENZFELD argues that being aware of and accepting these "liminal asymmetries" as well as explicitly naming them can help alleviate frustration and helplessness for both researchers and research participants.

Experiencing birth and death are also not ordinary experiences for most researchers. The lack of options to 'sufficiently' prepare for witnessing the death or birth of other people might be an explanation why some anthropologists identify a necessity or demand for some sort of "training" in preparation for fieldwork in such existential settings: For instance, ADRIENNE E. STRONG (2020) and MOLLY FITZPATRICK (2022) underwent training as doulas, i.e. a non-medical birth support person, before starting fieldwork on birthing and midwifery practices, and SCOTT STONINGTON (2020) and MENZFELD (2022) underwent training as an end-of-life doula and a voluntary terminal carer respectively prior to their ethnographic research on dying and end-of-life care. Training can help develop the right kind of sensitivity and self-confidence for encountering the beginnings and ends of life. Moreover, it can prepare us for fieldwork situations that might demand that we step out of the corner, out of the position of the observer. Becoming involved in settings of life and death – to assist, support, lend a hand and intervene – can be an inherently ethical demand in such settings, as it carries a different weight than involvements in less immediate life and death matters. The potential consequences of our actions, or inactions, tend to be significantly more pressing and irrevocable when it involves birth or death. Sometimes we act more than anticipated, which might cause us discomfort regarding our self-conception as anthropologists.

The demand to get involved in clinical and care work, to participate in daily tasks without having "proper" professional training, can not only be explained by the existential demands of giving birth or dying, but also emphasizes the fact that medical institutions, care homes, midwifery clinics, birthing centres and hospices are chronically understaffed and underresourced. In the contexts we discuss here, the lack of trained staff might quickly turn into a matter of immediate life and death – unlike in other contexts, in which the harmful effects of the privatization and underfunding of healthcare and the broader care sector materialize more slowly. STRONG, for example, refers to her motivation to train as a doula prior to fieldwork as "in the hopes of being useful" (2020: 18) in the Tanzanian clinic where she planned to conduct fieldwork. Besides concerns regarding sufficient personnel, her hope to be of use in the respective clinic hints at the sometimes-awkward position observing, waiting, chatting, scribbling ethnographers occupy in the diverging temporalities of medical settings amidst the rushing and waiting of nurses and doctors, patients and relatives. There is no easy role for anthropologists, who do not fit into the three common roles of the patient, the medical worker and the relative or visitor, and they may therefore appear as inappropriately occupying space and time (WIND 2008: 82f). The assumed need to be trained as a doula or terminal carer before fieldwork also points to implicit and explicit norms in these medical settings, which centre around expertise and formal knowledge. These are relevant not only regarding the question of *how* to intervene but also *whether* to intervene or not. While these questions depend to some degree also on whether one is allowed or feels able to intervene, to *not* intervene can also be a sign of expertise. Often the result of careful, expertise-driven and experience-based considerations, decisions to refrain from an intervention require a deep understanding of the matter at hand. This is as crucial for anthropologists as fieldworkers, as it is for midwives or doulas during birth (FITZPATRICK 2022; SKEIDE 2018) and terminal carers or palliative care professionals during people's dying (ANDRADE NEVES 2022; BORGSTROM, COHN & DRIESSEN 2020; MENZFELD 2022).

The contributions in this special issue pick up on recent discussions in anthropology which emphasize different approaches to "participation" that encounters at the beginnings and ends of life demand. Similar to ANNEKATRIN SKEIDE (2018), who reflects on the proximity of the roles of midwives/doulas and ethnographers as witnesses, MOLLY FITZPATRICK (2022) argues that being a "doula-ethnographer" while doing fieldwork on natural birth in Bali meant combining the very similar characteristics of both fields, such as empathy, understanding, listening or stepping back with one's own assumptions and assessments in order to foreground the birthing woman. At the same time, being able to assist legitimized FITZPATRICK'S presence in these settings and provided her with an affective understanding of what giving birth meant to the women she accompanied in Bali. More so, she argues that the existential, intimate and emotional nature of such experiences creates the need for ethnographers to go beyond mere presence and engage in an affective and embodied way. But FITZPATRICK also cautions that providing care as an anthropologist does not dissolve the discomfort one might feel as "witness" to such experiences – rather, ethical questions regarding our presence and our role need to be negotiated again and again, from moment to moment. In sum, she makes a strong plea for moving from a mode of "being-there" to a mode of "being-with" when doing research on birth. In the context of palliative care and dying, "being-with" has also been conceptualized as a

form of participatory presence, an active passiveness or entering a situation without an agenda. ANNELIEKE DRIESSEN, ERICA BORGSTROM and SIMON COHN (2021), for instance, discuss the importance and qualities of "being-with" when caring for people at their end of life – an important feature of palliative care that became disrupted and often impossible to maintain during COVID-19 lockdown measures.

Thinking of the onto-hierarchical differences between researchers and research participants at the end of life (MENZFELD 2022), MARCOS ANDRADE NEVES (2022) asks whether ethical preferences can outlive the people who make them. His article centres on the dilemma between acknowledging the importance of naming practices within political struggles for the right to assisted suicide and the anthropologist's responsibility in protecting research participants who – due to their death – will never have the opportunity to know how their stories will be told by the anthropologist. Based on his fieldwork on assisted suicide in the UK, Germany and Switzerland, ANDRADE NEVES argues that we need to consider the "afterlife reverberations" of our research – "the affects and expectations that ripple in the aftermath of a research participant's death from their research choices made in life" (2022: 18). Considering these, ANDRADE NEVES contends that it might be the anthropologist's responsibility to re-evaluate research participants' choices and opt for unnaming rather than naming practices. In his contribution, what is 'ethical' becomes hard to grasp and contested. The article sheds light on the situational and temporal aspects of research ethics, which – as we have argued above – make it difficult to attend to ethical questions in a standardized way, as often proclaimed in clinical settings.

Concluding remarks

Taken together, the contributions to this special issue illustrate that ethnographic explorations at the beginnings and ends of life raise crucial questions for anthropology's methodological "tool-kit" of pseudonymization, participant observation, self-reflexivity and positionality. They also highlight how ethics in anthropological research is always situative and negotiated, and, thus, transgresses clearly defined and neatly drawn definitions of most ethical boards and biomedical ethicists. In the existential moments of giving birth or dying, the presence of an ethnographer risks being perceived as awkward, inappropriate or unwelcomed – particularly in clinical settings, where anthropologists need to negotiate their roles and responsibilities not only with those birthing and dying, but also with clinical staff and within clinical routines, timelines and temporalities. These negotiations are evident also in settings that constitute alternative or complementary institutions to the clinic, such as the midwife-led birth clinic in Bali, the homes and hospices in Germany, or the semi-private spaces that facilitate assisted suicide in Switzerland.

As this special issue aims to maintain, the beginnings and ends of life serve as a magnifying glass – for ethnographic research and anthropological concepts, for questions concerning what 'ethical' means in these contexts, as well as for the political dimensions that run through these existential experiences. Access to maternal healthcare, as well as to alternatives to clinical care like midwife-led birthing centres, is as unequally distributed as access to competent palliative care at the end of life or the legal option and medical expertise for assisted dying. Giving birth and dying, as existential and universal as these experiences are, have, thus, inherent political dimensions. It is these which require us as anthropologists to remain critical and reflective of our doings, of the topics we choose to explore, the people we include in our research and our writing – keeping in mind how our doings potentially reverberate. The following contributions discuss these methodological and ethical issues and offer concepts that can be productively adapted to other research contexts. We hope that this special issue, although firmly grounded in the study of the beginnings and ends of life, will be an inspiration for researchers beyond this specific focus.

Notes

1 We use the term "white" in italics to point to the constructed nature of skin colour as a marker for differentiation and hierarchization (NDUKA-AGWU & HORNSCHEIDT 2010: 32f).

References

ABU-LUGHOD, LILA 1990. Can there be a feminist ethnography? *Women & Performance: A Journal of Feminist Theory* 5, 1: 7–27.

ADRIAN, STINE 2020. Stitching stories of broken hearts. Living response-ably with the technologies of death and dying at the beginning of life. *Australian Feminist Studies* 35, 104: 155–69.

ANDRADE NEVES, MARCOS 2022. Afterlife Reverberations: Practices of Un/naming in Ethnographic Research on Assisted Suicide. *Curare* 45, 2: 15–25.

AULINO, FELICITY 2019. *Rituals of Care. Karmic Politics in an Aging Thailand*. Ithaca: Cornell University Press.

BEHAR, RUTH 1996. *The Vulnerable Observer. Anthropology that Breaks Your Heart*. Boston: Beacon Press.

BEHAR, RUTH & GORDON, DEBORAH A. (eds) 1995. *Women Writing Culture*. Berkeley: University of California Press.

BENKEL, THOMAS & MEITZLER, MATTHIAS (eds) 2021. *Wissenssoziologie des Todes*. Weinheim: Beltz.

BIEHL, JOÃO 2001. Vita. Life in a zone of social abandonment. *Social Text* 19, 3: 131–49.

BORGSTROM, ERICA; COHN, SIMON & DRIESSEN, ANNELIEKE 2020. "We come in as 'the nothing.'" Researching non-intervention in palliative care. *Medicine Anthropology Theory* 7: 202–13.

BUCHBINDER, MARA 2021. *Scripting Death. Stories of Assisted Dying in America*. Oakland: University of California Press.

CHADWICK, RACHELLE JOY & FOSTER, DON 2014. Negotiating risky bodies. Childbirth and constructions of risk. *Health, Risk & Society* 16: 68–83.

CHAPARRO-BUITRAGO, JULIETA 2022. Debilitated lifeworlds. Women's narratives of forced sterilization as delinking from reproductive rights. *Medical Anthropology Quarterly* 36: 295–311.

CLARKE, ADELE E. & SHIM, JANET 2011. Medicalization and biomedicalization revisited. Technoscience and transformations of health, illness and American medicine. In PESCOSOLIDO, BERNICE A.; MARTIN, JACK K.; MCLEOD, JANE D. & ROGERS, ANNE (eds) *Handbook of the Sociology of Health, Illness, and Healing*. New York: Springer: 173–99.

CLARKE, ADELE E.; SHIM, JANET K.; MAMO, LAURA; FOSKET, JENNIFER RUTH & FISHMAN, JENNIFER R. 2003. Biomedicalization. Technoscientific transformations of health, illness, and US biomedicine. *American Sociological Review* 68, 2: 161–94.

COLEN, SHELLEE 1995. Stratified reproduction and West Indian childcare workers and employers in New York. In GINSBURG, FAYE D. & RAPP, RAYNA (eds) *Conceiving the New World Order: The Global Politics of Reproduction*. Berkeley: University of California Press: 78–102.

DAS, VEENA 2020. *Textures of the Ordinary. Doing Anthropology after Wittgenstein*. New York: Fordham University Press.

DAS, VEENA & HAN, CLARA (eds) 2016. *Living and Dying in the Contemporary World. A Compendium*. Oakland: University of California Press.

DAVENPORT, BEVERLEY ANN 2000. Witnessing and the medical gaze. How medical students learn to see at a free clinic for the homeless. *Medical Anthropology Quarterly* 14, 3: 310–27.

DAVIS, DÁNA-AIN. 2019. Obstetric racism. The racial politics of pregnancy, labor, and birthing. *Medical Anthropology* 38, 7: 560–73.

DAVIS, DÁNA-AIN & CRAVEN, CHRISTA 2016. *Feminist Ethnography. Thinking through Methodologies, Challenges, and Possibilities*. Lanham: Rowman & Littlefield.

DAVIS-FLOYD, ROBBIE 1992. *Birth as an American Rite of Passage*. Berkeley: University of California Press.

—— 1994. The technocratic body. American childbirth as cultural expression. *Social Science & Medicine* 38, 8: 1125–40.

—— 2019. Contemporary birth. A global overview. *Biomedical Journal of Scientific & Technical Research* 20, 3: 15121–5.

DRIESSEN, ANNELIEKE; BORGSTROM, ERICA & COHN, SIMON 2021. Ways of "being with." Caring for dying patients at the height of the COVID-19 pandemic. *Anthropology in Action* 28, 1: 16–20.

ENGELKE, MATTHEW 2019. The anthropology of death revisited. *Annual Review of Anthropology* 48, 1: 29–44.

FITZPATRICK, MOLLY 2022. From 'Being There' to 'Being With': Negotiating Affect and Intimacy while doing Ethnography at the Beginning of Life. *Curare* 45, 2: 37–50.

FOUCAULT, MICHEL 2003. *The Birth of the Clinic. An Archaeology of Medical Perception*. London: Routledge [orig. 1963].

FRASER, GERTRUDE J. 1995. *African American Midwifery in the South. Dialogues of Birth, Race, and Memory*. Cambridge, MA: Harvard University Press.

GAMMELTOFT, TINE & WAHLBERG, AYO 2014. Selective reproductive technologies. *Annual Review of Anthropology* 43: 201–16.

GARCIA, ANGELA 2016. Death as a resource for life. In DAS, VEENA & HAN, CLARA (eds) *Living and Lying in the Contemporary World. A Compendium*. Oakland: University of California Press: 316–28.

GINSBURG, FAYE D. & RAPP, RAYNA (eds) 1995. *Conceiving the New World Order. The Global Politics of Reproduction*. Berkeley: University of California Press.

GOTTLIEB, ALMA 1995. The anthropologist as mother. Reflections on childbirth observed and childbirth experienced. *Anthropology Today* 11, 3: 10–14.

HARAWAY, DONNA 1988. Situated knowledges. The science question in feminism and the privilege of partial perspective. *Feminist Studies* 14, 3: 575–99.

HARDING, SANDRA (ed) 2004. *The Feminist Standpoint Theory Reader. Intellectual and Political Controversies*. New York: Routledge.

HERTZ, ROBERT 1960. *Death and the Right Hand*. London: Routledge [orig. 1907].

INHORN, MARCIA 2021. Infertility, in vitro fertilization, and fertility preservation. In HAN, SALLIE & TOMORI, CECÍLIA (eds) *The Routledge Handbook of Anthropology and Reproduction*. London: Routledge: 217–32.

JAIN, S. LOCHLANN 2013. *Malignant. How Cancer Becomes Us*. Berkeley: University of California Press.

JORDAN, BRIGITTE 1993. *Birth in Four Cultures. A Crosscultural Investigation of Childbirth in Yucatan, Holland, Sweden, and the United States*. Long Grove: Waveland Press [orig. 1978].

KAUFMAN, SHARON R. 2005. *And a Time to Die. How American Hospitals Shape the End of Life*. Chicago: University of Chicago Press.

—— 2015. *Ordinary Medicine. Extraordinary Treatments, Longer Lives, and Where to Draw the Line*. Durham, NC: Duke University Press.

KAUFMAN, SHARON R. & MORGAN, LYNN M. 2005. The anthropology of the beginning and ends of life. *Annual Review of Anthropology* 34: 317–41.

KRAWCZYK, MARIAN & RICHARDS, NAOMI 2021. A critical rejoinder to "Life's end: Ethnographic Perspectives". *Death Studies* 45, 5: 405–12.

LAYNE, LINDA. 2003. *Motherhood Lost. A Feminist Account of Pregnancy Loss in America*. London, New York: Routledge.

LOCK, MARGARET 2002. *Twice Dead. Organ Transplants and the Reinvention of Death*. Berkeley: University of California Press.

MARKS, HARRY M. 2012. Chemonotes. *Social History of Medicine* 25, 2: 520–39.

MARTIN, EMILY 2001. *The Woman in the Body. A Cultural Analysis of Reproduction*. Boston: Beacon Press.

MBEMBE, ACHILLE 2003. Necropolitics. *Public Culture* 15, 1: 11–40.

MENZFELD, MIRA 2022. Liminal Asymmetries. Making Sense of Transition Dynamics in Relations with Dying Persons. *Curare* 45, 2: 26–36.

MULLINGS, LEITH 2021. The necropolitics of reproduction. Racism, resistance, and the Sojourner Syndrome in the age of the movement for Black Lives. In HAN, SALLIE & TOMORI, CECÍLIA (eds) *The Routledge Handbook of Anthropology and Reproduction*. London: Routledge: 106–22.

NAHMAN, MICHAL. 2016. Reproductive tourism, through the anthropological "reproscope". *Annual Review of Anthropology* 45: 417–32.

NDUKA-AGWU, ADIBELI & HORNSCHEIDT, ANTJE LANN 2010. Der Zusammenhang zwischen Rassismus und Sprache. In NDUKA-AGWU, ADIBELI & HORNSCHEIDT, ANTJE LANN (eds) *Rassismus auf gut Deutsch. Ein kritisches Nachschlagewerk zu rassistischen Sprachhandlungen*. Frankfurt a. M.: Brandes & Apsel Verlag GmbH: 11–59.

NIEDER, LUDWIG & SCHNEIDER, WERNER (eds) 2007. *Die Grenzen des menschlichen Lebens. Lebensbeginn und Lebensende aus sozial- und kulturwissenschaftlicher Sicht*. Münster: LIT Verlag.

OAKLEY, ANN 1981. Interviewing women. A contradiction in terms? In ROBERTS, HELEN (ed) *Doing Feminist Research*. London: Routledge: 30–61.

RAPP, RAYNA 1999. *Testing Women, Testing the Fetus. The Social Impact of Amniocentesis in America*. New York: Routledge.

REHSMANN, JULIA 2018. Confined live(r)s. Self-infliction and arbitrary survival in the German transplant system. *Anthropological Journal of European Cultures* 27, 2: 45–64.

—— 2019. Dancing through the perfect storm. Encountering illness and death in the field and beyond. In STODULKA, THOMAS; DINKELAKER, SAMIA & TAJIB, FERDIANSYAH (eds) *Affective Dimensions of Fieldwork and Ethnography*. Cham: Springer: 189–200.

———— 2021. Lists in flux, lives on hold? Technologies of waiting in liver transplant medicine. In VINDROLA-PADROS, CECILIA; VINDROLA-PADROS, BRUNO & LEE-CROSSETT, KYLE (eds) *Immobility and Medicine. Exploring Stillness, Waiting and the In-between.* Singapore: Palgrave Macmillan: 15–37.

———— 2022. Failing livers, anticipated futures and un/desired transplants. *Anthropology & Medicine* 29, 1: 92–106.

ROSALDO, RENATO 1993. Grief and a headhunter's rage. In ROBBEN, ANTONIUS C. G.M. (ed) *Death, Mourning, and Burial. A Cross-Cultural Reader.* Oxford: Wiley Blackwell: 156–66.

ROSE, NIKOLAS 2007. *The Politics of Life Itself. Biomedicine, Power, and Subjectivity in the Twenty-First Century.* Princeton: Princeton University Press.

RUDRAPPA, SHARMILA 2012. Working India's reproductive assembly line. Surrogacy and reproductive rights? *Western Humanities Review* 66, 3: 77–101.

SALLNOW, LIBBY ET AL. 2022. Report of the Lancet Commission on the Value of Death. Bringing death back into life. *The Lancet* 399: 837–84.

SCHEPER-HUGHES, NANCY 1993. *Death without Weeping. The Violence of Everyday Life in Brazil.* Berkeley: University of California Press.

SIEGL, VERONIKA 2018a. Aligning the affective body. Commercial surrogacy in Moscow and the emotional labour of Nastraivatsya. *TSANTSA. Journal of the Swiss Anthropological Association* 23: 63–72.

———— 2018b. The ultimate argument. Evoking the affective powers of "happiness" in commercial surrogacy. *Anthropological Journal of European Cultures* 27, 2: 1–21.

———— 2019. Uneasy thankfulness and the dilemma of balancing partiality in surrogacy research. In STODULKA, THOMAS; DINKELAKER, SAMIA & TAJIB, FERDIANSYAH (eds) *Affective Dimensions of Fieldwork and Ethnography.* Cham: Springer: 87–96.

———— forthcoming 2023. *Intimate Strangers. Commercial Surrogacy in Russia and Ukraine, and the Making of Truth.* Ithaca: Cornell University Press.

SKEIDE, ANNEKATRIN 2018. Witnessing as an embodied practice in German midwifery care. In KRAUSE, FRANZISKA & BOLDT, JOACHIM (eds) *Care in Healthcare. Reflections on Theory and Practice.* Cham: Springer: 191–209.

SOOM AMMANN, EVA & REHSMANN, JULIA 2022. Tinkering am Lebensende. Wie die Pflege das Sterben in der Institution gestaltet. In CADUFF, CORINA; AFZALI, MINOU; MÜLLER, FRANCIS & SOOM AMMANN, EVA (eds) *Kontext Sterben.* Zürich: Scheidegger & Spiess: 112–22.

STACEY, JUDITH 1988. Can there be a feminist ethnography? *Women's Studies International Forum* 11, 1: 21–7.

STAVRIANAKIS, ANTHONY 2019. *Leaving. A Narrative of Assisted Suicide.* Oakland: University of California Press.

STONINGTON, SCOTT 2020. *The Spirit Ambulance. Choreographing the End of Life in Thailand.* Oakland: University of California Press.

STRONG, ADRIENNE E. 2020. *Documenting Death. Maternal Mortality and the Ethics of Care in Tanzania.* Oakland: University of California Press.

VAN DER GEEST, SJAAK 2007. Is it possible to understand illness and suffering? *Medische Antropologie* 19, 1: 9–21.

VAN HOLLEN, CECILIA C. 2003. *Birth on the Threshold. Childbirth and Modernity in South India.* Berkeley: University of California Press.

WACKERS, GER 2016. Recursive health care structures and choice in the manner of our dying. An auto-ethnographic account. *Qualitative Health Research* 26, 4: 452–65.

WIND, GITTE 2008. Negotiated interactive observation. Doing fieldwork in hospital settings. *Anthropology & Medicine* 15, 2: 79–89.

WOJTKOWIAK, JOANNA & MATHIJSSEN, BRENDA 2022. Birth and death. Studying ritual, embodied practices and spirituality at the start and end of life. *Religions* 13, 9: 820–6.

ZIVKOVIC, TANYA 2021. Lifelines and end-of-life decision-making. An anthropological analysis of advance care directives in cross-cultural contexts. *Ethnos* 86, 4: 767–85.

JULIA REHSMANN Dr., is a social anthropologist and postdoctoral fellow at the Bern University of Applied Science and the University of Bern. As part of the interdisciplinary research project "Settings of Dying" (project no. 188869) she is currently conducting ethnographic research on palliative care in Switzerland, exploring how expertise and gender shape end-of-life care. For her PhD research, situated in the research project "Intimate Uncertainties" (SNSF project 149368), she explored liver transplants in Germany and examined how the high-tech field of transplant medicine is interwoven with moral and intimate questions about 'lives worth saving'. Together with Sarah Hildebrand, Gerhild Perl and Veronika Siegl she published the book "Hope", a collaboration between social anthropology, photography and literature.

Bern University of Applied Sciences, Department of Health Professions, Nursing Research
Murtenstrasse 10, 3008 Bern, Switzerland
julia.rehsmann@bfh.ch

VERONIKA SIEGL Dr., is a social anthropologist and gender studies scholar. She is currently a Postdoc.Mobility Fellow of the SNSF and located at the University of Vienna, as a Senior Research Fellow, and the University of Cambridge, as a Visiting Scholar. Her work focuses on questions of ethics, inequality and autonomy in the context of medicine, technology and the body. In her current project, she explores how the category of "life" is negotiated in the context of prenatal testing and selective abortions in Austria. For her dissertation, she scrutinized how morals and values are employed to make sense of, judge, legitimise and govern the intimate and affective relations produced in the sphere of commercial surrogacy in and beyond Russia and Ukraine. Based on this research, her book "Intimate Strangers" will be published with Cornell University Press in 2023.

University of Vienna, Department of Social and Cultural Anthropology
Universitätsstraße 7, 1010 Vienna, Austria
veronika.siegl@univie.ac.at

Afterlife Reverberations

Practices of Un/naming in Ethnographic Research on Assisted Suicide

MARCOS FREIRE DE ANDRADE NEVES

Abstract Can ethical choices outlive the people who make them? In order to explore this question, this article draws on ethnographic research on transnational assisted suicide to question afterlife implications of practices of un/naming, particularly the use of anonymisation and pseudonyms. Assisted suicide is organised around a specific politics of naming that animates its fight for social and political recognition but which contradicts anthropology's once long-standing disposition towards anonymity as a form of protecting research participants. This dissonance creates a situation where one of anthropology's main tools of protection risks jeopardising the political struggles and fight for recognition of the same people it seeks to protect. Against this background, this reflection argues that empirically researching death and dying requires an additional sensitivity to un/naming practices. Thus, I propose the notion of afterlife reverberations, that is, the affects and expectations that ripple in the aftermath of a research participant's death from their research choices made in life.

Keywords anonymity – assisted suicide – research ethics – pseudonym – un/naming

Introduction

"We need a British Brittany Maynard", the words echoed inside the large library room where about 30 people gathered for the assembly general meeting of a UK-based charity that advocates for increased awareness of end-of-life choices. These words, uttered by a member of the organisation, resonated with several of the people attending the meeting, most of whom agreed with the proposition while others seemed confused by it. Brittany Maynard's case was well-known in the right-to-die debate after she made her own story public with the intention of pushing for further legalisation of aid-in-dying in the United States. Maynard, who was diagnosed with terminal glioblastoma when she was 29 years old, decided to move from her home state of California to Oregon, where she died using the provisions of the state's Death with Dignity Law. "We need a high-profile case", the voice continued, "I don't want anyone to die, less so young people, but it's a way to draw attention and push for legislative change". At the time Maynard's case became public, five US states allowed some form of aid-in-dying, and the attention generated by her case gave motion to legislative debates across the country,

which culminated in the legalisation of aid-in-dying in several other states, including her home state of California.

As anthropologist NAOMI RICHARDS (2014) points out, the right-to-die debate in the UK has been dominated by high-profile cases that generate attention by emphasising individual suffering. Despite taking place in a different jurisdiction, Maynard's case followed a similar logic: by exposing her struggles with glioblastoma and her journey towards aid-in-dying, Maynard was able to influence public and legislative debates in the US and overseas. The legalisation of aid-in-dying is a deeply contentious issue that is prone to political, legal, medical, religious, and moral controversies. In this troubled environment, people's individual suffering is often invested with political and moral meanings (RICHARDS 2014: 17) that can animate such controversies and push for institutional response. Thus, the implications of having a "British Brittany Maynard" are twofold: on the one hand, it indicates the ability of high-profile cases to attract public attention and effect change, and, on the other hand, it highlights the importance of making one's own name and trajectory public. Over the years, several litigations on the right-to-die revolved around individuals who made their names, stories, and suffering known to the wider public (MENEZES 2011; RICHARDS 2011; WARD 2015), a move that acts to personalise the right-to-die debate by attaching names to it and, consequently, life stories. This holds the potential to attract greater public and political sensibility to the issue. Thus, Maynard's case speaks to a politics of naming that sits at the heart of the right-to-die debate, holding the potential to raise public awareness, stir controversies in different domains, and push for legal and legislative changes.

When the suggestion of having a "British Brittany Maynard" was brought forward, I was observing the meeting as part of my fieldwork on transnational assisted suicide[1], which I carried out from 2015 to 2017 in Germany, Switzerland, and the United Kingdom. As the meeting unfolded and the discussion about the need for a high-profile case continued, I noticed the irony of making notes about a meeting on the centrality of naming while unnaming everyone involved in this discussion. Whereas anthropologists have long relied on practices of unnaming, such as pseudonymisation and anonymisation, to protect their research participants, this irony left me wondering how to reconcile the need for protection in a research field that relies on naming to push for social and political legitimation. The question underlying this thought was how to compose an ethnographic description that protects the people involved in the research when our main tool of protection risks undermining their own fight for recognition. Whereas the need for naming or the impossibility of unnaming in certain research contexts have already been widely discussed (NELSON 2015; THOMSON 2021; WALFORD 2018), ethnographic research on end-of-life complicates this further since many participants will not live to see the research outcome—and, as a result, will not experience the consequences of their decisions regarding anonymity.

As JULIA REHSMANN and VERONIKA SIEGL argue in the introduction to this special issue, exploring beginnings and ends of life can pose new questions that challenge "long-held traditions and taken-for-granted research practices"

(2022: 5), including un/naming decisions. In this article, I delve into this unplanned irony of unnaming everyone during a meeting on the importance of naming to reflect on methodological and ethical questions raised by navigating a research space that is situated at the margins between life and death. This is a space where the anthropological imagination of what constitutes ethical practice needs to be reevaluated and rearranged in accordance to a new set of commitments and expectations that continues to reverberate and have real life implications after the death of the people who made them. In such cases, where participants are unable to respond or react to the research outcome, ethical commitments need to be reshaped to include possible implications that continue to unfold after their death; implications that continue to affect the researcher, the deceased, as well as their family members and friends.

Over the course of my research, I have met several individuals involved directly or indirectly in aid-in-dying, such as campaigners, professional assistants, and people who are applying for assisted suicide and may or may not opt to carry out the procedure at some point. I asked each participant to sign an informed consent form where, among other things, they had to indicate their wish to be anonymised or have their real names used. Against the background of this highly contentious issue that often relies on high-profile cases to advance its agenda, most participants opted for the latter option. Most participants, however, were also aware of the likelihood that they would no longer be alive to see how their names were employed. They would not be able to protest how their names were used or to comment on the final version of the text. They would no longer be alive to see the implications of a decision they made while living, but which would continue to reverberate and produce effects after their death. To explore the uneasy dimension of research ethics that emerge in between life and death, this article proposes the notion of afterlife reverberations, that is, the concerns, affects, and expectations that ripple in the aftermath of a person's death from their research choices made in life. To explore afterlife reverberations is to question whether ethical choices can outlive the people who made them, challenging an imaginary of research ethics that was consolidated upon the expectation of reciprocity, protection through anonymity, and, fundamentally, of being alive.

If being alive is taken for granted in anthropology's imaginary of research ethics, what are the afterlife reverberations triggered by research spaces where death and dying are no longer something to be avoided, but someone's ultimate goal as the result of an intricate process that can be empirically apprehended? In order to explore afterlife reverberations in this special issue dedicated to ethical and methodological challenges of doing ethnographic research at the beginnings and ends of life, the following reflection will first set out its larger framework. This introduces the broader context of assisted suicide and the possibility of empirically researching and experiencing the death of others that its legalisation facilitated. Subsequently, I will address the so-called name problem of assisted suicide, exploring the centrality of naming practices as a key factor in attracting public attention and effecting change through legislative and/or legal pathways. I will base my reflection on the naming problem on the trajectories of research participants who shared their life stories with me, in particular Margot and Paul[2], and use their experiences, struggles, and successes as a guide for this narrative. Finally, I will discuss afterlife reverberations as another layer of ethical reflection that emerges from doing ethnography at the margins between life and death.

Researching the Death of Others

"You're the most important person in Margot's life here", I heard Dr Preisig saying to me as Margot was offering her final goodbyes. We were in a flat in the outskirts of Basel, Switzerland, when moments after this statement Margot died while holding my hand. The flat was spacious yet empty, comfortable but impersonal. Its white walls were flooded with natural light coming through the windows that overlooked a rather grey industrial zone. And as the sound of multiple voices in the room gave way to a deep silence, Margot took her final breath, dying the kind of death she expected and hoped for—one she considered to be safe, fast, and painless, taking place before her quality of life deteriorated any further. While Dr Preisig was checking Margot's pulse, I was simply there, standing next to Margot and trying to hold back my tears. Margot was pronounced dead while we were still alive, waiting for the police to come to deal with the aftermath of her dying. For people involved with aid-in-dying in Switzerland, this is routine. The police always come afterwards to ensure that the death occurred due to assisted suicide, which can be legally performed, thus discarding any possibility of foul play. And while this situation was unfolding around me, that is, while the police and the state prosecutor were verifying all documents of Margot's application process and the coroner checked her body, I was trying to reconcile my roles as someone who was both being *there* and *with*. As a researcher I was *there* witnessing what seemed to be a rich research event, but I was also being *with* Margot, my friend who died holding my hand just a few minutes before.[3]

Switzerland is often the main destination of people applying for organised assisted suicide worldwide, particularly due to the coupling of a favourable legal environment and the work of several specialised organisations, at least three of which accept non-Swiss citizens and residents as members. The friction caused by this local legislation with the mostly unfavourable legal environment beyond Swiss borders often leads to the transnational mobility of people who leave their home countries to achieve their aspirational death in Switzerland. Defined by the anthropologist MARA BUCHBINDER (2021: 6), aspirational death refers to the "aesthetic, affective, and ethical preferences that inform orientations to dying as a matter of personal choice and careful choreography". In the present context, aspirational death is employed to reflect on notions of good death that are articulated within each individual situation—the best death possible given the circumstances. Crossing national borders to achieve an aspirational death was precisely Margot's case when she travelled from Germany to Switzerland to receive Dr Preisig's assistance. Despite its prominence, Switzerland is one piece in the complex tapestry of aid-in-dying that emerged in the 20th century and has gained special traction since the 1980s. At this time, several European jurisdictions started to consider the legalisation of aid-in-dying, be it through judicial or legislative paths. Since then, several European countries have legalised some form of aid-in-dying, such as the Netherlands (in 1984 by court ruling, followed by state law in 2002), Belgium (2002), Luxembourg (2009), and Austria (2022).

Notwithstanding this legal trend, medical aid-in-dying is not a new phenomenon. In fact, as FRANCES NORWOOD (2018: 461) argues, medical professionals have been helping people to die at least since the beginning of modern medicine. What is new is not the practice itself but its incorporation into state law, including the possibility of non-medical assistance. It is against this background that, as noted by BUCHBINDER (2021), death becomes something that can be legally done rather than something that merely happens. The gradual emergence and consolidation of aid-in-dying also gave rise to new research spaces where the production of specific kinds of death can be empirically captured, including, but not limited to, palliative care and assisted suicide (ANDRADE NEVES 2020; BUCHBINDER 2021; LEMOS DEKKER 2018a, 2018b, 2020; MENEZES 2004; NORWOOD 2006, 2007). For instance, Margot's aspirational death was not one that would just happen by chance, but one that needed to be carefully orchestrated and actively produced through human and pharmaceutical intervention in an organised setting. The circumstances of her aspirational death, which involved a lengthy application process, ended up facilitating the possibility of participant observation throughout the entirety of this process and during the procedure itself (ANDRADE NEVES 2020). Yet the emergence of such research spaces where people cross the border between life and death also poses a challenge to an imaginary of research ethics formulated around the expectation of life and living and not the anticipation of death and dying.

When we accompany the death of others in such research spaces, what tools are available to us to create an ethical research environment that protects participants while being attentive to the real-life implications of their wishes? For instance, reflecting on her experience of doing research at the end of life, MARIAN KRAWCZYK (2017: 2) points to the ambivalence of having an "ethically robust" process of consent while simultaneously questioning the appropriateness of her own presence in the field. "I have come to

believe the ethical considerations regarding the presence of the researcher in such situations", she writes, "should not only include the participant's capacity to provide consent but should also be informed by the relationships that have developed between the researcher and the participant" (ibid.). These research relationships are developed and shaped against the background of different anticipations of death and dying—that is, different expectations between researcher and participant regarding the temporality of their own death and dying. In research situations that take place in close proximity to death and dying, how effective is anthropology's usual ethics repertoire of informed consent and practices of unnaming? How does one provide protection to participants through unnaming when their names are crucial elements in their own fight for recognition and political legitimation? Essentially, how can anthropological research be ethical when the foundations of what we assumed to be ethical principles are turned upside down by empirically researching the death of others?

The Name Problem

The effectiveness of high-profile cases like Brittany Maynard's relies on the articulation of individual suffering into the public sphere, where its visibility can elicit affects and give renewed motion to public debates. As RICHARDS (2014: 17) argues, "personal stories are now instrumentalized, by both 'sides' of the right-to-die debate, in order to generate media coverage and public sympathy for a cause". In fact, the reliance of high-profile cases on publicising individual suffering and personal stories is underlined by a politics of naming that is vital in the larger right-to-die debate and which mirrors the choices regarding anonymity made by most participants in my research. While conducting fieldwork, I asked research participants to sign an informed consent form in which one of the questions was devoted to un/naming preferences. It questioned: "The participant wishes to remain anonymous in any publications based on the interviews/participation in the research", followed by "yes" and "no" boxes. To my initial surprise, partly due to a naive and unreflective disciplinary expectation towards unnaming, most participants crossed "no", indicating they did not wish a pseudonym. In the conversations that followed, they often reaffirmed their preference to have their real names employed. Whereas a politics of naming sits at the heart of the larger right-to-die debate and reverberates with individual choices regarding naming preferences, it contradicts anthropology's long-standing principle of anonymising research participants as a form of protection.

One of said high-profile cases was Paul Lamb's, a former builder who got paralysed from the neck down in the aftermath of a car accident. Several years after the accident, Lamb joined Tony Nicklinson in a legal fight for the legalisation of voluntary euthanasia in the UK. Nicklinson, who suffered from locked-in syndrome, died six days after an unfavourable High Court ruling (RICHARDS 2014). After his death, Nicklinson's former solicitor and his widow contacted Paul Lamb and invited him to join the case, which they intended to continue. At first, they suggested he could join the case anonymously as "L" to protect his privacy. As Lamb recounted to me, he initially agreed to be disguised as L, which made him feel like a "James Bond character". Shortly afterwards, however, the solicitor approached him again to ask whether he would be willing to "come out in the open", claiming that everyone thought L was a fictitious character. As Lamb was unsure about what "coming out in the open" entailed, the solicitor speculated that probably some people would contact or come to see him. Once again, Lamb agreed, and while fearing the worst, he ended up feeling surprisingly overwhelmed by demonstrations of support. His and Nicklinson's case gained traction and, although rejected again, helped to inform the right-to-die debate in the country.

Paul Lamb and I met during my fieldwork at his home in Leeds. When I visited him prior to the interview, he signed an informed consent form in which he indicated his wish to have his real name used. He was no longer willing to be L. Lamb's preference reflected his previous trajectory from anonymity to publicity, from having his identity concealed to having his real name disclosed both in the legal proceedings and the media. What right did I have to disguise Lamb once again, wrapping his identity under another pseudonym, when his political and legal fight was based precisely on him leaving L behind

and publicly assuming his own identity? As JULIA VORHÖLTER (2021: 15) argues, concealing the identities of research participants has been a central ethical principle of anthropological research, but its main goal of not harming research participants risks overshadowing the complexity and moral ambiguity of anonymity. VORHÖLTER argues that a balance needs to be found between respecting a participant's interests and wellbeing and anthropology's high ethical standards. In Lamb's case, where "coming out in the open" was a crucial step in his trajectory, unnaming him under the guise of protection would be a violent act that undermines his ongoing political struggle and jeopardises his own personal interests.

Lamb, alongside the vast majority of participants in my research, opted against the use of pseudonyms to represent them in the final text, paving a situation where the standard disciplinary practice of unnaming participants clashed with their own preferences to be identified. Upon reviewing all informed consent forms and reflecting on my process of establishing consent, the feeling of protection I was expecting to accomplish for myself and participants alike was met by the realisation that the tools I had to offer went against their own instruments for social and political recognition. In retrospect, similarly to the experience described by KRAWCZYK (2017: 2), while I also perceived my process of consent as "ethically robust", its guiding assumptions did not take into consideration the specificity of this field, thus failing to anticipate the dilemmas and implications of a field where some participants are expected to die during the research. I was relying on informed consent forms and frequent conversations to understand the living and dying circumstances of each participant and to place their individual preferences into the wider context of the research. As the informed consent form becomes synonymous with the principle of respect for autonomy (HOEYER & HOGLE 2014: 350), it ends up creating an "illusion of the ethical" (CANNELLA & LINCOLN 2007: 316). It creates a false expectation that main ethical concerns can be addressed and resolved within the margins of a standard document that reflects a specific idea of what research ethics looks like; an illusion that obfuscates ethics as a relational, complex, and ongoing process that requires constant attentiveness to the ordinary (DAS 2015). After all, as LAMBEK (2015: 34) puts it, being attentive "includes being responsive, being awake, being engaged in and with the world".

According to WEISS and MCGRANAHAN (2021), "[t]he use of pseudonyms is partially that of an inherited disciplinary custom deployed unreflectively". Indeed, my default position of what constituted an ethical research practice clashed with the politics of naming of assisted suicide, turning the expectation of ethical practice into the frustration of ethical violence—the enforcement of certain ethical standards over the participants' own interests. While discussing futuring trans* in Pakistan, the anthropologist OMAR KASMANI (2021: 97) notes that "acts of naming and unnaming, be they partially, ambiguously, or situationally adopted as individual, multiple, or collective iterations, constitute manifest labours of affective world making". Indeed, following KASMANI's reflection and applying it to my research context, acts of un/naming needed to be resolved individually against the larger background of the research, balancing the politics of naming of assisted suicide with different interests and real-life implications. Whereas requests for anonymising were immediately respected, requests for the use of real names were considered case-by-case.

For instance, returning to the description of Margot's death, the complexity and ambiguity of un/naming practices can be further explored. In her informed consent form, Dr Preisig opted "no" for having a pseudonym, while Margot signalled "yes", but added a note: she wanted me to use her first name as pseudonym. Margot's choice was a compromise shaped by political and personal factors, as she wanted to contribute personally to what she saw as an ongoing political struggle for the recognition and legalisation of assisted suicide, while minimising the possibility of exposing her family. In this sense, Margot's choice encapsulates an interplay between her own anticipation of possible afterlife reverberations in regards to her family and the political dimension of assisted suicide, where naming plays a fundamental role. In Dr Preisig's case, similarly to Paul Lamb's, it would be difficult to anonymise her, as she is a public figure who often takes part in media debates on assisted suicide. Her involvement with

aid-in-dying and professional engagement with the issue made her request to use her real name easy to follow, as anonymising her would conceal her years of political struggle and activist work. To anonymise her properly, the organisation she founded and the city where it is based would have to be anonymised as well—as it was the only organisation of its kind in Basel at the time.

Also Margot's individual decision needed to be placed in a collective context, against which it became clear that the information she provided over the course of the research would potentially lead to her identification and, consequently, to the identification of her family. Margot, however, would no longer be able to re-evaluate her choice, as she knew from the outset of our relationship that she would likely die a death by appointment before the conclusion of the research. The name problem of assisted suicide, thus, is twofold: Firstly, assisted suicide operates following a publicising logic, where conveying identity is fundamental to advance its political agenda and fuel its struggle for recognition. This logic, however, challenges anthropology's ethical apparatus, as the discipline's main tool to secure protection and disguise identity undermines the participants' struggles for legitimation. Secondly, in a research context where participants often die a voluntary and planned death, the afterlife implications of their preferences expressed in life need to be taken into consideration, as they will no longer be able to change their minds and reconsider their choices. This leads to the fundamental issue my article is concerned with: doing ethnography on death and dying requires additional sensibility to practices of un/naming, as participants' choices need to be evaluated against the anticipation of their death and ethical commitments need to be expanded to include its possible consequences—their afterlife reverberations.

Afterlife Reverberations

While guaranteeing anonymity has become a standard practice in anthropology, we employ it by making assumptions that are often misguided or incomplete. Even though Margot asked me to use her first name, I did not. Margot is a pseudonym I created after her death. As WEISS and MCGRANAHAN (2021) suggest, practices of naming and unnaming, in particular the use of pseudonyms, have real life implications that go beyond methodological issues. Margot's real first name alone would not be able to convey her identity. It was a common name after all. However, in conjunction with other elements of her life story, such as place and year of birth, professional trajectory, and family background, people close to her could easily assume her identity. For instance, it could be suspected easily by her family, who expressed no desire to know the details of her death—a wish that Margot respected in life, but risked jeopardising in death. Margot had already anticipated possible afterlife reverberations when she made what she considered a good compromise between personal and political dimensions in her choice regarding the use of her first name. However, she would no longer be around to (re)evaluate whether this compromise actually worked to her liking. She would no longer be able to deal with the impact that her death and her taking part in the research might have on her family. With her death, the ethical commitments established between us changed, as it was now up to me to assess possible implications that her death and my narration of it might have on her family—an assessment Margot would not be able to evaluate or protest against.

The ambivalence of making a final decision about un/naming a deceased person that may either validate or go against their preferences expressed in life is a key ethical challenge of doing ethnographies at the end of life, as the proximity of death rearranges our ethics landscape to take into account the impact of someone's death on decisions communicated in life. In her book about stories of aid-in-dying in the US, MARA BUCHBINDER (2021: 17) argues that there is "something discomforting about using stories of one person's tragedy for professional gain". This discomfort, however, is compounded when combined with unnaming decisions that often need to go against the participant's preferences, particularly in the aftermath of their dying. Whereas, as BUCHBINDER (2021) notes, their death and tragedy are a source of professional gain for the researcher, the retelling of their stories holds the potential to shift the debate on a topic that not only is highly controversial, but also illegal in most jurisdictions across the world. However discomforting this process may feel, ethnography holds the potential to both contribute to and fuel a wider debate by providing an intimate account of death and dying. If we employ pseudonyms unreflectively as a sign of disciplinary inertia, are we not, as SARA SHNEIDERMAN (2021) suggested, undermining "ethnography's potential as an instrument of recognition?"

Un/naming choices are crucial and have real life consequences. As JASON THROOP (2014) pointed out, our ethical commitments tend to change according to un/naming decisions. Would I still be willing to write about Margot's life if I used her real name instead? Would I enjoy the same intellectual enthusiasm to explore intimate moments in life, or the intimacy of closely being with her in dying, if the audience was aware of her identity? In the aftermath of my research, when translating several life and death stories into a final narrative, I respected everyone's wishes for disguising their identity. When it came to individual preferences to employing real names, however, I reflected on the potential real-life consequences of their individual choices, keeping in mind that individual decisions can have collective effects. This is precisely what the notion of afterlife reverberation entails, the consideration of ethnographical concerns, expectations, and affects that ripple after someone's death and may affect the research and the lives of those who stayed alive in ways that were previously unforeseen. To consider afterlife reverberations is to open oneself to vulnerability and uncertainty, embarking on a journey that seeks to reconcile the lived past with the unfinished present from affects that continue to blossom and reverberate after death.

Margot was eager to tell her life story before her appointment in Basel, and I was eager to hear it. And over the course of several interactions, which included joining her for her last dinner, she did it. She composed a narrative about her own life, one that articulated her trajectory with her desire to die a specific kind of death. Her story was now mine to recount, but––and she was well aware of this––she would no longer be able to hear my version of it. How can I create a narrative that is based on life stories conveyed to me by people who knew they would not be able to verify it? If, on the one hand, to consider afterlife reverberations is crucial to reflect on the impact of a participant's death during the research, on the other hand such reverberations may have different intensities according to the relationships that were developed over the course of the research. Intimacy, thus, is an indispensable element to calibrate afterlife reverberations. For instance, in the aftermath of Margot's assisted suicide, I left the organisation's flat on foot. I wanted to walk to the closest train station and board a train to the city. I felt the need to get some fresh air and be alone while I tried to mend the pieces of everything that had happened that morning—and the months before. But as I walked to the train station, the funeral home car drove past me and honked, offering a ride. I wanted to be alone but could not resist the irony of crossing paths with Margot once again and accepted the offer.

When I arrived in the city, I had nowhere to go. My flight back home would only depart a few hours later. Lacking better ideas and emotionally exhausted, I decided to go to the nearest fast food place. As I hung my coat over the chair, I felt an envelope in my pocket that I knew was there but had forgotten existed. Margot gave me this envelope just before her procedure but asked me not to read it until she was gone. I treasured the envelope in my pocket, somewhat conflicted about it. I was curious to read it, yet I knew that reading it meant Margot was dead. When I felt the envelope, everything came back to my mind, all memories of our brief but dear friendship. I was no longer able to hold back the tears I had successfully hidden all this time. When Margot and I first met, we did not know each other's faces. She had sent me a photo of herself by post, but it did not arrive in time. So I made a suggestion to her: when I arrive at the restaurant, I will raise my green cell phone to the air, so if you see it, let me know. She did see it and waved back at me. The envelope was also green, the same green. So was the ink she had used to write the letter.

"To intimate", beautifully argues LAUREN BERLANT (1998: 281), "is to communicate with the sparest of signs and gestures". In her final message to me, Margot made a simple choice that took us full circle right back to our first contact. She communicated this intimacy not with words, but with colour and affect. She gave another life to our friendship after her death, bringing back memories and making me reflect on our past trajectory and future possibilities, imbuing in me a sense of responsibility that highlighted even further the importance and challenges of considering afterlife reverberations. At the time of her procedure, although I was the only one present who knew Margot from before, we by then had known each other for just a few months. In the weeks and months that followed our first meeting, Margot would regularly call me and send me letters. At the time, she was still applying for the procedure, so her death by appointment was something she anticipated but was unsure of. More than knowing how she wanted to die, Margot knew until when she wanted to live. She drew a line between what was acceptable to her and what was not, indicating that if this line was about to get crossed, she would act to avoid it. She would schedule her appointment and begin her final journey to Basel. After we met for the first time and our relationship unfolded, Margot realised she wanted me to be there with her as she released the flow of the lethal medication down the cannula and into her vein; as she walked into the flat and out of her life. Doing intimacy during encounters that include a person's transition from life to death can place the researcher in distinct roles and lead to different waves of afterlife reverberations. The intimacy I developed with Margot over the course of several encounters and interactions throughout the research intensified the afterlife reverberations from her death, as I had to reflect on her ethical choices by anticipating its future implications; a reflection process that was calibrated by our relationship and the kind of intimacy we developed.

Our friendship unfolded over the course of her death process, in between her initial application and the final procedure. When the latter took place, I was not just there, observing everyone's actions and witnessing her final moments. I was *with* her—not only as an indication of physical proximity, but also, and fundamentally, of a particular affective dimension that emerged out of doing intimacy in the context of contrasting life and death temporalities, of contrasting finitudes. While addressing the context of palliative care during the COVID-19 pandemic, DRIESSEN, BORGSTROM & COHN (2021: 17) emphasise the importance of palliative professionals conveying a perception of "being with" the patients as a key aspect of doing intimacy and building trust. Being with, in this sense, implies conveying a sense of genuine interest that goes beyond the professional obligation of being there. While, on the one hand, being with relies on intimacy and trust building, on the other hand, as MOLLY FITZPATRICK writes in this special issue, being with also demands a constant negotiation of the ethics of such relationships. As a mode of engagement that can be both "uncomfortable and riddled with complex ethical considerations" (FITZPATRICK 2022: 2), being with is an intricate form of care that is shaped by intimacy. And this intimacy of being with, in turn, affects the stakes and intensity of afterlife reverberations.

My relationship with Margot evolved within the framework of my research on assisted suicide, where we also established the terms of her participation and her conditions for consent—including in regards to naming. While this is customary in ethnographic research, what is specific to this context is the anticipation of her death by appointment, which brings with it the certainty that her ethical choices would outlive her—and that she would have no opportunity to review, contest, or even regret them. The conditions of her participation would likely be affected by her death, rearranging the ethical configuration to include new commitments, responsibilities, and expectations. My ethical commitment with Margot was both professional and personal, as a researcher and friend, as someone who was there and with.

Final Remarks

The legalisation of different forms of aid-in-dying has enabled the emergence of research spaces in which a specific form of death can be legally done and, thus, empirically apprehended as a complex process that involves a whole range of different actors. One of these research spaces, organised assisted suicide, is a highly controversial subject whose legal quality is frequently being debated and contested in different jurisdictions. To advance its pro-legalisation agenda, people involved in the right-to-die debate often follow the logic of so-called high-profile cases, where individual suffering is articulated away from the private and into the public sphere. Brit-

tany Maynard is one of such high-profile cases, and so is Paul Lamb. They opted to publicise their names and individual trajectories in order to give traction to the public conversation—Lamb, for instance, made the choice of ceasing to being L and assumed his own name. Underlying the logic of high-profile cases lies a politics of naming that is crucial to eliciting public affects, stirring controversies, and pushing for legislative change.

Thus, when it comes to political and legislative struggles of assisted suicide, acts of naming can be crucial to advance the debate. But whereas assisted suicide relies on naming to fuel the debate, anthropology often follows a long-standing preference for unnaming research participants with the aim of protecting their identity and respecting their privacy. This dissonance assembles the background to this article: the kind of ethical sensibility that emerges when assisted suicide, with its naming preference, and anthropology, with its unnaming imperative, meet in a research space located at the intersection of life and death. In this text, I have reflected on my experience of doing ethnography on the end-of-life to explore the ethical implications of this dissonant encounter. I argue that the discipline's primary tool for protection can exert ethical violence by jeopardising the struggle for recognition of the very people it seeks to protect. While this implication can be shared by other fields and research areas, I have directed attention to the specificity of assisted suicide as a research field: the likelihood that participants will die a voluntary death over the course of the research, which raises questions on accountability and rearranges the ethical commitments established between participant and researcher during life. In the foreground, lies the question of whether ethical choices can outlive the participants who made them.

In order to explore this question, I proposed the notion of afterlife reverberations to address the continuous affects and effects that ripple in the aftermath of a participant's death, where ethical choices need to be reevaluated under the light of their possible implications to the researcher, to participants' family and friends, as well as to the participants themselves. While afterlife reverberations need to be considered in research contexts where participants die an aspirational death, the intensity of such reverberations is adjusted by the intimacy established between researcher and participants. At the risk, as SHNEIDERMAN (2022) has warned, of poisoning anthropology's potential as a tool for recognition, being open to afterlife reverberations also means rethinking and reordering the ethics landscape of anthropology to account for the implications of death and dying during the research and its aftermath. Whereas the individual dies, the ethical subject lives on. But following a participant's death, their ethical preferences expressed in life need to be considered and reflected upon under a different light. When carrying out ethnographic explorations at the end of life, I propose that afterlife reverberations be explicitly discussed with research participants, anticipating the possibility that their deaths may trigger previously unforeseen dilemmas that hold the potential of reshaping their agreed upon ethical commitments.

Acknowledgments

My thanks to Julia Rehsmann, Veronika Siegl, Mira Menzfeld, and Molly Fitzpatrick for their thorough reading and critical input throughout this process. I am also grateful to Ehler Voss, Janina Kehr, and the anonymous reviewers for their feedback, as well as to Simon Patterson for his careful reading and valuable criticism. I would also like to thank Erika, Margot, and Paul for contributing to this reflection by sharing their life stories and for welcoming me into their lives.

Notes

1 Throughout this article, I have chosen to use the term assisted suicide to refer to the specific form of aid-in-dying described here, while aware of the politics of language animated by the term suicide. The term assisted suicide puts emphasis on the self-administered dimension of the practice, contrasting it with physician-administered procedures, such as euthanasia. These procedures, despite their mutual dis/connections, usually enjoy different legal status within the same jurisdiction. For instance, whereas assisted suicide can be legally performed in Switzerland, euthanasia remains a criminal offence. Therefore, clarity is key to avoid ambiguity. To quote an interlocutor who was discussing her views on terminology, "we don't like the term, but assisted suicide tells you what it is". While the association with suicide can be controversial, the term assisted suicide directs the focus to self-administration,

which is crucial to avoid a shadow of suspicion that could lead, in the extreme, to assistants being criminally prosecuted.

2 Whereas the text reflects on un/naming practices through anonymity choices, it should be noted that the discussion can be further expanded onto other naming practices, such as the differential use of first and last names. As MARGOT WEISS suggests, textual representation through first or last names often indicates a split between interlocutors and scholars, thus reproducing "disciplinary hierarchies" (2021: 949). In the present text, the use of first or last name in the case of interlocutors was decided following the interplay of anonymity choices, possible afterlife reverberations, intimacy, as well as narrative roles. Using Dr Preisig's last name and title, for instance, was thought as a way of highlighting her role in this dynamic as a medical professional.

3 For a thorough discussion between being there and with see MOLLY FITZPATRICK's contribution in this special issue.

References

ANDRADE NEVES, MARCOS 2020. Protecting Life, Facilitating Death: The bureaucratic experience of organized suicide assistance. *Medicine Anthropology Theory* 7, 1: 158–166.

BERLANT, LAUREN 1998. Intimacy: A special issue. *Critical Inquiry* 24, 2: 281–288.

BUCHBINDER, MARA 2021. *Scripting Death. Stories of Assisted Dying in America*. Oakland, California: University of California Press.

CANNELLA, GAILE S. & LINCOLN, YVONNA S. 2007. Predatory vs. Dialogic Ethics: Constructing an Illusion or Ethical Practice as the Core of Research Methods. *Qualitative Inquiry* 13, 3: 315–335.

DAS, VEENA 2015. What does ordinary ethics look like?. In LAMBEK, MICHAEL; DAS, VEENA; FASSIN, DIDIER & KEANE, WEBB (eds) *Four lectures on ethics: anthropological perspectives*. Chicago: Hau Books: 53–125.

DRIESSEN, ANNELIEKE; BORGSTROM, ERICA & COHN, SIMON 2021. Ways of 'Being With': Caring for Dying Patients at the Height of the COVID-19 Pandemic. *Anthropology in Action* 28, 1: 16–20.

FITZPATRICK, MOLLY 2022. From 'Being There' to 'Being With': Negotiating Affect and Intimacy while doing Ethnography at the Beginning of Life. *Curare* 45, 2: 37–50.

HOEYER, KLAUS & HOGLE, LINDA F. 2014. Informed Consent: The Politics of Intent and Practice in Medical Research Ethics. *Annual Review of Anthropology* 43, 1: 347–362.

KASMANI, OMAR 2021. Futuring Trans* in Pakistan: Timely Reflections. *TSQ: Transgender Studies Quarterly* 8, 1: 96–112.

KRAWCZYK, MARIAN 2017. Approaching death: Informed consent and research relationships at the end of life. *Medicine Anthropology Theory* 4, 2. http://www.medanthrotheory.org/article/view/5603/ [31.08.2022].

LAMBEK, MICHAEL 2015. Living as if it mattered. In LAMBEK, MICHAEL; DAS, VEENA; FASSIN, DIDIER & KEANE, WEBB (eds) *Four lectures on ethics: anthropological perspectives*. Chicago: Hau Books: 5–51.

Lemos Dekker, Natashe 2018a. "I do want euthanasia, but not now." Timing a request for euthanasia with dementia in the Netherlands. http://somatosphere.net/2018/i-do-want-euthanasia-but-not-now-timing-a-request-for-euthanasia-with-dementia-in-the-netherlands.html/ [20.04.2022].

—— 2018b. Moral frames for lives worth living: Managing the end of life with dementia. *Death Studies* 42, 5: 322–328.

—— 2020. Anticipating an unwanted future: euthanasia and dementia in the Netherlands. *Journal of the Royal Anthropological Institute* 27: 815–831.

McGranahan, Carole 2021. The Truths of Anonymity: Ethnographic Credibility and the Problem with Pseudonyms. https://americanethnologist.org/features/collections/rethinking-pseudonyms-in-ethnography/the-truths-of-anonymity-ethnographic-credibility-and-the-problem-with-pseudonyms/ [20.04.2022].

Menezes, Rachel 2004. *Em busca da boa morte: antropologia dos cuidados paliativos.* Rio de Janeiro: Editora Fiocruz/Garamond.

—— 2011. Demanda por eutanásia e condição de pessoa: reflexões em torno do estatuto das lágrimas. *Sexualidad, Salud y Sociedad* 9: 137–153.

Nelson, Rebecca 2015. Pseudonyms 2.0: How Can We Hide Participants' Identities When They're on Pinterest? https://savageminds.org/2015/10/08/pseudonyms-2-0-how-can-we-hide-participants-identities-when-theyre-on-pinterest/ [30.08.2022].

Norwood, Frances 2006. A hero and a criminal: Dutch *huisartsen* and the making of good death through euthanasia talk in The Netherlands. *Medische Antropologie* 18, 2: 329–347.

—— 2007. Nothing More To Do: Euthanasia, General Practice, and End-of-Life Discourse in the Netherlands. *Medical Anthropology* 26, 2: 139–174.

—— 2018. The New Normal: Mediated Death and Assisted Dying in the United States. In Robben, Antonius C. G. M. (ed) *A companion to the anthropology of death.* Hoboken: Wiley: 461–475.

Rehsmann, Julia & Siegl, Veronika 2022. The Beginnings and Ends of Life as a Magnifying Glass for Ethnographic Research: Introduction to the Special Issue. *Curare* 45, 2: 5–14.

Richards, Naomi 2014. The death of the right-to-die campaigners. *Anthropology Today* 30, 3: 14–17.

Shneiderman, Sara 2021. Collapsing Distance: Recognition, Relation, and the Power of Naming in Ethnographic Research. https://americanethnologist.org/features/collections/rethinking-pseudonyms-in-ethnography/collapsing-distance-recognition-relation-and-the-power-of-naming-in-ethnographic-research/ [20.04.2022].

Thomson, Marnie Jane 2021. Names are Problems: For Congolese Refugees, for the Humanitarian System, and for Anthropological Writing. https://americanethnologist.org/features/collections/rethinking-pseudonyms-in-ethnography/names-are-problems-for-congolese-refugees-for-the-humanitarian-system-and-for-anthropological-writing [30.08.2022]

Throop, Jason 2014. Friendship as Moral Experience: Ethnographic dimensions and ethical reflections. *Suomen Antropologi: Journal of the Finnish Anthropological Society* 39, 1: 68–80.

Vorhölter, Julia 2021. Anthropology Anonymous? Pseudonyms and Confidentiality as Challenges for Ethnography in the Twenty-first Century. *Ethnoscripts* 23, 1: 15–33.

Walford, Geoffrey 2018. The impossibility of anonymity in ethnographic research. *Qualitative Research* 18, 5: 516–525.

Ward, Amanda 2015. *Who Decides? Balancing competing interests in the Assisted Suicide debate.* Glasgow: University of Glasgow.

Weiss, Erica & McGranahan, Carole 2021. Rethinking Pseudonyms in Ethnography: An Introduction. https://americanethnologist.org/features/collections/rethinking-pseudonyms-in-ethnography/rethinking-pseudonyms-in-ethnography-an-introduction/ [20.04.2022].

Weiss, Margot 2021. The Interlocutor Slot: Citing, Crediting, Cotheorizing, and the Problem of Ethnographic Expertise. *American Anthropologist* 123, 4: 948–953.

Manuscript received: 22.04.2022
Manuscript accepted: 31.08.2022

MARCOS FREIRE DE ANDRADE NEVES | Dr. phil., is a researcher and lecturer at the Institute of Social and Cultural Anthropology at Freie Universität Berlin, where he is affiliated with the Research Area Medical Anthropology | Global Health. He currently holds a DAAD PRIME Fellowship at the University of Edinburgh, where he conducts a research on the circulation of sodium pentobarbital, focusing on medico-legal entanglements that are triggered as it travels across different jurisdictions. His previous research was an ethnography on the transnational circulation of people, pharmaceuticals, and technologies in the context of organised assisted suicide, focusing mainly on Germany, Switzerland, and the United Kingdom. He published the book "Por Onde Vivem os Mortos" (UFRGS University Press) and directed the documentary "Torotama: A Grave Matter".

Freie Universität Berlin / University of Edinburgh
Thielallee 52, 14195 Berlin
marcos.freire@fu-berlin.de

Liminal Asymmetries

Making Sense of Transition Dynamics in Relations with Dying Persons

MIRA MENZFELD

Abstract The article presents one option for an anthropologically informed understanding of onto-hierarchical particularities that can characterize and shape relationships between non-dying persons (e. g. researchers) and dying interlocutors. The article draws on research with responsive and conscious persons who 1) suffer from a terminal illness, 2) have been informed about their terminal prognosis, and 3) regard their diagnosis as reliable information about their own dying. The classic Turnerian ideas of *threshold* and *transition dynamics* are applied to make sense of *liminal asymmetry* as an important factor that permeates research relations with consciously dying persons and can sometimes create challenging situations during fieldwork. Liminal asymmetries are characterized by at least three dimensions. First, as dying persons are in a 'betwixt-and-between' state, they often desire liminal companionship and guidance when dying. (Persons who are not terminally ill are inherently incapable of adequately fulfilling the role of liminal guide or companion because they are not in a state of betwixt-and-between.) Second, the experience of hierarchy is crucial, as the dying have privileged access to a mode of being that the non-dying have not yet entered. Third, as another existential hierarchy, dying persons – having accepted a terminal diagnosis as a reliable statement about their presence and future – usually consider their state of being, agency, and vitality to be less privileged than that of non-dying persons. By acknowledging liminal asymmetries as formative for experiences of dying, we gain an additional tool for understanding research situations in which liminal asymmetries are directly or indirectly thematized. The article describes two exemplary fieldwork scenarios to illustrate the types of situation identified as arenas for negotiating the (im)possibilities of liminal companionship and liminal guidance, as well as capability-related hierarchies.

Keywords dying – participant observation – liminality – liminal asymmetry – terminal illness

Introduction

On entering into a relationship with an aware-of-dying[1] person – that is, a person in a phase of life that they themselves identify as an irreversible process of dying – researchers are meeting someone who is willing to spend part of the last weeks of their life with someone they barely know. This comes with a responsibility; there is a particular requirement for politeness and a heightened necessity not to annoy a person who is terminally ill, often exhausted, and sometimes rather desperate. Despite the researcher's best efforts, there is still a risk of appearing tiresome or even overburdening a dying interlocutor (MENZFELD 2022; 2018a; APPLETON 2004; PALGI & ABRAMOVITCH 1984; see also CHATTERJI 2016, WOODTHORPE 2011, RIESSMAN & MATTINGLY 2005, BEHAR 1996). Through an anthropological lens, this article describes one way of understanding some possible sources of exhaustion and annoyance for the interlocutor that can also cause researchers to feel insecure.

Field research with people who are dying means working with people whose current mode of existence necessarily remains fundamentally incomprehensible – at least unless the researcher is acutely and terminally ill. On the one hand, this does not essentially distinguish end-of-life participant observation from other ethnological work contexts; after all, anthropologists are constantly trying to understand people and circumstances whose being and doing they cannot always comprehend from an emic point of view. On the other hand, when working with the dying, the characteristically anthropological residual omission in the field can appear especially drastic. Interlocutors who have been informed about their terminal prognosis and have internalized this as a statement about their personal future and state of being are especially likely to have a strong sense of their situation as radically different from that of the researcher. Some dying persons experience anger, envy, and deep feelings of injustice when they realize that they probably have only a short time to live; in contrast, the researcher and other non-dying persons may assume that they have far more time (MENZFELD 2021). In addition, long periods of conscious silence, partial inability to communicate, and communication-inhibiting fatigue are to be expected among dying interlocutors, and researchers must also endure and recognize the particular nonverbal expressiveness of these situations. 'Coming in as the nothing' – as BORGSTROM ET AL. (2020) recently characterized the attitude adopted by some palliative carers (not only) in UK contexts as an alternative to overactive or curative action logics – is perhaps neither task-appropriate nor possible for researchers. However, the underlying idea – to avoid giving unsolicited advice, interfering uninvited, or simply causing undue annoyance to the dying person – is worth considering as a useful aspiration for research attitudes, including settings beyond palliative care (see also FITZPATRICK 2022; ANDRADE NEVES 2022, both in this volume).

But why is that so? Are there specific features of the relationship between dying and non-dying persons that explain why it seems so easy to overstep the line during contact and why different professionals[2] explicitly or instinctively conceptualize a respectful approach to the terminally ill as 'coming in as the nothing'? In explaining the hidden or open hierarchies between aware-of-dying persons and non-dying persons, are we missing something by focusing on the general vulnerabilities of the terminally ill – on death anxiety, emotional turmoil in the face of dying, or the general tragedy of mortality?

I would like to draw attention to a dimension of dying that, in my opinion, can be a source of misunderstandings and problems if it remains an unconscious co-factor in relationships between non-dying persons and dying people. I explore what I call *liminal asymmetry* by resorting to the classic anthropological concept of liminality, which will be explained in detail below (TURNER 1967, 1974; VAN GENNEP 2006[1909]). In particular, I explicate the frequent absence of eye-level companionship and guidance within the liminal phase of terminal illness. This absence can make dying persons feel abandoned and stressed, and cannot be compensated for by non-dying persons: not by the most dedicated physicians, not by the most skilled therapists, not by the most loving relatives, and certainly not by anthropological researchers. Unless understood and reflected, a lack of liminal guidance and companionship can be frustrating, leaving both sides – dying and non-dying alike – with feelings of helplessness. However, simply being aware that liminal asymmetries are no one's fault but are rooted in fundamentally different modes of liminal or non-liminal states of being can help both sides to understand and accept their individual and mutual limitations. More particularly, the awareness can open up a space for dealing constructively with possible thematizations of liminal asymmetries by accommodating them within the research relationship. In this article, I present and analyse two examples from my long-term fieldwork with dying persons in Germany to illustrate some concrete situations in which the issue of liminal asymmetry may be assumed to occur.

Liminal Guidance and Companionship: A Need That Non-Dying Persons Cannot Meet

Although dying is widely acknowledged as a prime example of a liminal phase (see for example SCHRÖDER 1986; KAUFMAN & MORGAN 2005; THOMPSON 2007), research on dying tends to treat this as a standalone insight – which is a pity, as it has sufficient explanatory potential to be considered much more than a commonplace. I argue that some potentially stressful or even research-inhibiting situations occur not only during research-related contact with dying persons but also during other contact between non-dying and dying people. The reasons for this can be more precisely identified by paying due regard to TURNER's (1964, 1967, 1969, 1974) understanding of liminal situations.

As I explain in detail elsewhere (MENZFELD 2018a) and as addressed and conceptualized in a slightly different way by thanatologists rooted in sociology (WALTER 2007; WALTER ET AL. 2012; SEALE 2004),[3] a demand for what TURNER (1974) called *communitas* can be observed from time to time in terminally ill persons. Terminally ill persons may experience moments of deep happiness on finding a support group where they can exchange experiences about their situation. Sometimes, they benefit from knowing that an old friend or relative is suffering from an incurable illness at the same time as they are, affording opportunities for comradeship. In contrast, dying persons who have no contact with others who are terminally ill[4] may feel existentially lonely, different from everyone else, and misunderstood – even those who are constantly surrounded by caring relatives, doctors, nurses, and friends.

Such feelings cannot simply be explained away by characterizing the existential loneliness of dying merely as some kind of cultural fault or as a means of denying death, as some classic tropes of thanatology suggest (most prominently perhaps ARIÈS 1976 and 1981; see also BECKER 1973; GIDDENS 1991).[5] Instead, to understand what dying people may long for but cannot get from non-dying persons, it helps to look at what TURNER (1964, 1967, 1969, 1974) identified as the core characteristics of liminality. Turner contended that people who experience a liminal transformation find themselves in a betwixt-and-between state of ontological indifference; that liminality is characterized by a change of status involving an initiation; and that people in this liminal phase have very different options and restrictions on agency than those in a non-liminal state.

All of these aspects of liminality inform contemporary aware dying in European biomedical contexts (see also REHSMANN & SIEGL 2022) in the following way. Dying people live with the ontological particularity of being aware that their future is very limited; they receive this message through a unique initiation that usually involves a diagnosis statement from a biomedical specialist (who is assumed to be capable of making reliable prognoses in this regard). Moreover, dying people receive specialized medical care (e. g. palliative rather than curative), are excluded from certain financial transactions (e. g. bank loans), and are no longer expected to work the same hours as before. They are also encouraged to think about their last will and to engage in final conversations with those close to them, et cetera (see MENZFELD 2018a for a contextualized account of shifts in agency options and activity limits for dying persons).

However, Turner also identified elements that are *not* entirely met when the dying process is initiated by a biomedical expert as crucial in liminal situations; these include:

- initiation by an already initiated person;
- guidance throughout the liminal phase from an already initiated guide;
- conventionalized communitas among liminal companions;
- a conventionalized procedure of personal reintegration that the liminal person herself experiences although transformed through liminality.

(TURNER 1964, 1969, 1974; see also VAN GENNEP 2006 [1909])

In exchanges with persons who are consciously dying and who are initiated through the normalized procedure (i. e. diagnosis by a biomedical expert whose judgement is considered reliable), we meet people who have had no opportunity to talk to someone who has already experienced dying. As those who have already experienced the liminal phase of dying are already dead, they are not available to give advice to the newly initiated.[6] The dying person is not initiated by someone who has successfully completed the initiation process but by a specialist who assesses their physical condition and, based on this assessment, draws conclusions about their current and future ontological and action-related status in terms of capacity (i. e. whether the person is living or acutely dying, needs rest, or is able to perform daily routines as usual). While every biomedical prognosis refers only to probabilities and likelihoods – that is, assumptions about how a disease might manifest in a particular individual and how quickly it might kill them – the constitutive speech act of communicating a terminal diagnosis and the associated proceedings and requirements provoke a massive shift in how they see themselves and are seen by others, in the possibilities and limits of action, and in the emergence of new uncertainties and limitations.

It also becomes clear that *communitas* is uncommon; when dying persons are deliberately brought together, it is often for reasons of care management (e.g. in a palliative care unit or a hospice) rather than to encourage engagement with others in the liminal phase of dying. Non-dying people may even view spontaneous alliances between dying persons with suspicion or worry that contact between terminally ill people might increase the likelihood of sadness and despair (MENZFELD 2018a). It is not entirely normal for dying people to seek advice or contact with other dying persons; no cultural script suggests that dying people should seek the company of other dying people or envisages bringing dying persons into contact with each other. This clearly sets dying apart from other liminal phases, such as becoming a mother, which affords myriad opportunities for advice and contact (e.g. pregnancy yoga, birth preparatory courses). Although some prognoses indicate that seeking connections with fellow sufferers may be a trend among dying persons (WALTER 2017, 2003), we have not (yet) found evidence of any commonly shared assumption that it is good and normal for dying persons to socialize with others in a similar situation.

Among other concerns, the reintegration phase is confusing for many dying persons in terms of belief. Even among those who cultivate a strong belief in a personal life after death, the nature of personal reintegration cannot necessarily be regarded as reliable knowledge. Plainly speaking, dying persons cannot be sure they will experience some form of reintegration after passing away, and while some hold firm beliefs in this regard, many assume there will be no reintegration after the body dies.

The absence of liminal guidance and companionship and the uncertain prospects for reintegration can cause extreme discomfort. One can imagine similar levels of discomfort in other liminal situations. For example, some women would prefer to give birth for the first time under the guidance of someone who is not only a specialist but has also experienced childbirth herself. Similarly, young persons may experience initiation to adult life as adverse without liminal companions, and so on. In the liminal phase of dying, these missing features may cause stress. Keeping that in mind, encounters in the field, such as the two described below, can be seen in a new light.

Many of the dying interlocutors I grew close to described particular ways of responding to liminal differences (see also MENZFELD 2018a), leading me to a re-reading of Turner. Both of the situations described below occurred during fieldwork I undertook with dying persons in Germany between 2013 and 2016. I have chosen not to characterize either of my dying interlocutors in terms of their diagnosis, as this is unnecessary for understanding their situation. In addition, they were reluctant to be defined by their disease, and I regard it as a gesture of respect not to reduce them posthumously to a predominantly biomedical framing.

Konstantin

It was a rainy autumn evening in 2014. My interlocutor Konstantin, a married engineer aged 56 years, had agreed to see me despite feeling a little short of breath and tired that day. I went to his house without a second thought because I knew that he favoured conversation – despite the potential for exhaustion – rather than boredom and overthinking. More than once, he had told me that 'being part of all your lives means I'm still part of everything'. As he said this, he pointed at me and at his children, who were present at the time, but also at the blabbering TV. Konstantin often joked about his diagnosis; he allowed himself to cry, when he felt so inclined, in the company of his relatives. He was very busy preparing his last Christmas celebration and never ceased to be interested in his neighbours' smallest everyday problems or the latest political news. In short, Konstantin was the ideal image of someone who remains happy, joyful, and self-controlled to the very end.

Yet, like many aware-of-dying persons, he had his moments of deep anger and loneliness. When I entered his room on that rainy autumn evening, I instantly sensed that his glance seemed different from what I recalled of my previous visits. He sat partly upright in his bed; his face was still, his jaw slightly clenched, and he barely greeted me. I grabbed a chair and sat down by his bed. I said 'Hello' and asked how he felt. Konstantin did not indulge in flattering words or superficial politeness but simply answered 'Not well'. I nodded and sat silently beside him. Usually, our meetings would start with lighter conversation, but he apparently had no need for light conversation that day.

After a little while, Konstantin said, slowly, 'You know what's going on? Everything falls apart. I fall apart here. I watch myself falling apart. You do not know what this means'. During that last sentence, his eyes met mine. He did not seem angry or sad – just very, very serious. I looked back at him, touched by the seriousness and openness and nodded slowly. He said 'The problem is – you all think you understand. I also thought that once. But you do not [understand]'. I took some time to respond, because I felt a little shy; then I said 'Would you want us to understand you better? Maybe you can explain what we do not *get*?' Konstantin smiled kindly and answered 'I do not think this is possible. But that is just how it is'. He closed his eyes, and we were just present next to each other – him following his private thoughts or getting some rest, and me thinking about what he had said.

When Konstantin opened his eyes again, he asked me to get some juice and wanted to chat a little about what he called 'the tradition of groundless incompetence' of the local municipality in failing to build houses and community areas that do not look like they hate their own town 'because why else would they drown each little corner in concrete and ugly architecture?' His wife joined us a little later, and we chatted for about two hours in what seemed an easy-going atmosphere. When it was time for dinner, and I offered to leave this part of the day to him and his wife, Konstantin agreed. While his wife went to prepare an evening snack for him, Konstantin said a special goodbye to me: 'About our conversation when you came; you're not the problem [if you don't get everything that I experience]. Actually, I like it better this way, because if you were to get it [my experience] from the inside, you would all soon be lying here next to me'.

What first appears to be a contradictory tension – the initial wish to be understood and the awareness that this wish is not realizable in relations with non-dying persons – becomes more understandable if interpreted as an expression of Konstantin's longing to be understood by other dying persons rather than as a statement of non-dying persons' inability. In fact, he is not simply mourning the fact that nobody could ever understand what he is going through but recontextualizes his feelings by adding that anybody who *could* understand him would necessarily be dying too. In his last sentence, Konstantin echoes a statement that I heard increasingly when I began to develop research relationships with dying persons over a period of weeks or months. This leads me to assume that at least some aware-of-dying persons possess a strong sense of the limits of non-dying persons' comprehension of what life is like during the process of dying. Other interlocutors made similar comments when disappointed that no doctor could tell them how they would feel the next day, or when they struggled to find out whether it was normal to often feel sad in their situation or whether this form of depression required treatment, or when they received well-meant advice from their children to meet up one last time with old friends with whom they no longer had any contact, or even when they had just had a nice, easy-going chat with their partners. In short, demarcation statements of this kind highlight the difference between the dying and the non-dying and arise in a wide range of situations.

I assume that in statements such as Konstantin's last words to me at that meeting, there is a hint of an emic awareness of the liminal asymmetry between dying and non-dying persons. This awareness can be reflected practically in (among other things) the urgent feeling of being misunderstood by non-dying people, pointing indirectly (and sometimes directly) to the fact that non-dying people cannot actually guide or help the dying through the dying process. A mode of being that includes knowing that one has no more than a few months (at most) of a future or a life differs radically from anything that a non-dying person faces.[7] Even we establish a connection, dying persons themselves sometimes point out that radical difference between the dying and the non-dying.

Judith

The second situation I would like to introduce arose during a visit to a care institution. Judith, a divorced 66-year-old former taxi driver, had decided to move to an institution after she realized that living alone at home was becoming increasingly difficult for her. Her story, like Konstantin's, illustrates the experience of liminal asymmetries between oneself (as a dying person) and others who are not yet dying. Judith's story also shows how things can change when the people around you actually 'get' what dying means.

I had not visited Judith during the Christmas holidays, but I came to her room in January to see how she was and whether she was doing well in the small hospice. I was a bit worried that she might not like it there because, when she was test-living there to see whether she would find it comfortable to spend her last weeks in such an institution, there were conflicts with two of the nurses. In particular, Rudi – a carer she did not like and considered impolite – seemed to have become something of an in-house enemy, not least because she responded to his assumed rudeness with snappy comments of her own.

Judith also had reservations about talking to psychological counsellors and even to the younger doctors who were responsible for her medication and well-being. She was very compliant in respect of the doctors' recommendations, but she suffered from what she referred to as a dependence on 'little children right from university who mean the best but know nothing', which on some days included myself as a then-young researcher.[8] In expressing these views, she offended more than one of the professionals who were caring for her, and surely at least some of her friends, whom she clearly regarded as unable to understand her situation (although not as childlike, given their age or life experience). According to Judith, 'It is not enough for them that they are healthy and I am not; they also want me to tell them that they understand everything so they do not feel shut out or something [...] But that would only make *them* feel good; it would not be honest'.

Judith often felt lonely and once even complained, half-jokingly, that 'there is no Brockhaus [a lexicon on all matters of general knowledge] to look up what all this [dying] will be like'. At the same time, she strongly rejected advice and expressions of empathy from those who did not share her mode of living as a terminally ill person. To cope with this specific aspect of loneliness, she tended to read everything about dying (written by other dying persons) that she could get her hands on. For instance, she was a huge fan of Wolfgang HERRNDORF's (2013) book and his blog about his experience of dying from a glioblastoma. She also reported feeling very inspired and 'seen' when she read Christoph SCHLINGENSIEF's (2009) diary about his own process of dying of lung cancer.

When I entered her room on that January day, Judith appeared to be flourishing despite an obvious and apparently dangerously rapid loss of weight over the holidays, indicating that her physical condition may have worsened. As soon as I closed the door, Judith informed me excitedly that she had made contact with another resident at the facility who lived just down the hall. She had met him two days before Christmas Eve in the small park visible from the window of her room. She made a point of telling me that while he might not be the most handsome man, he was a person she could 'really talk to'. Although her new friend was much younger than her, he seemed to be one of the very few people that Judith could explicitly accept as an equal partner in conversation. Spontaneously, she characterized her relationship with her new friend as follows: 'If there's someone who knows what it feels like ... That's better'. After meeting her new friend, being misunderstood all but vanished from the list of topics that she regularly addressed. Although they rarely seemed to talk explicitly about the actual situation of dying, the mere fact that they were both going through a similar experience seemed comforting. This brought them closer together, and they accepted each other's company and advice despite rarely allowing anyone into their lives or permitting physical proximity.[9] One of the last things that Judith said about being annoyed by carers was the following: 'Since I found him [her new friend], I am not alone anymore, and honestly, I am less annoyed [by people who annoyed me before]'.

More than once, I noted in Judith's expressions and actions a very palpable enactment of missing liminal opportunities. She wanted to be guided by someone who had been through all the things she was currently dealing with, and if the only available guidance was to be found in books, she would at least read those books. She wanted to be in the company of people who shared her situation, who could really understand her, who would offer her a form of communal experience. Interestingly, the person Judith finally viewed as an equal was not of the same age, educational background, or socioeconomic status.

He was younger, more educated, and better off in economic terms, but she still saw him as an equal because he was also dying. Judith admitted that, since meeting him, she had what she longed for: a friend who understood the situation in which she found herself. Viewed through the Turnerian lens of transition(al) dynamics, Judith clearly had a history of bringing up and suffering from liminal asymmetries but found relief once she had a liminal companion.

Judith and Konstantin: Experiencing Liminal Asymmetries

In narrating these particular encounters with Judith and Konstantin, I want to stress two things. First, it is not easy to be in a liminal state when there is no liminal guide to turn to. Initiation into the dying process is usually performed by an uninitiated expert without any deeper insight into how it feels to be aware of one's own dying. Starting there, the trend continues, as most of the people around a dying person are not yet dying themselves. This can cause feelings of unease, of being misunderstood and clueless, and even of loneliness, sometimes resulting in a sense of existential abandonment during a transformative situation that cannot always be adequately alleviated by encounters with well-meaning, caring, or specialized persons, even those with psychological training. No one is to blame for this situation; the dilemma is typical of other experiences of chronic illness but is especially palpable in the case of dying. No matter how hard they try, non-dying persons cannot comprehend the full meaning and experience of liminality in dying. Even dying persons who say they have been cared for in the best possible way cannot deny that, at least sometimes, the company and guidance of a person who understands what they are feeling would be ideal or perhaps even necessary.

Second, I want to stress that some dying persons *do* actively look for ways of dealing with possible feelings of liminal abandonment and the crucial differences between themselves and the non-dying. Although rarely encouraged to do so (and perhaps even discouraged from doing so by non-dying persons), some dying persons actively pursue opportunities for exchange across the entire spectrum of liminal communi-

tas or look for liminal guidance in the writings of those who have been where they are now. Judith's story is an example of a dying person whose transition from being lonely to being accompanied by a new friend crucially influenced her view of her own dying process and her feelings about her life's ending. It is important to emphasize that these individual orientations towards liminal communitas and companionship are not what SEALE (2004) called *confessional deaths* (i. e. self-revelations in front of an audience that includes non-dying persons) and cannot be framed as a desire to share one's own dying experiences openly – for example, in social networks (WALTER ET AL. 2012). Interlocutors like Judith and Konstantin do not want to display their embeddedness in the social networks of the living; in fact, they do not want to make their dying public at all. While they yearn for guidance and/or companionship, they do not long to share their experiences with a larger non-liminal audience; they want contact with others whose onto-hierarchical specificities align with their own. To put it another way, they find their own ways of dealing with liminal asymmetries. The concept of *liminal asymmetries* helps to explain why Judith feels so much more comfortable as soon as she makes a friend of a very specific kind – another dying person – and why Konstantin declares so strongly that nobody around him could really understand his specific situation unless they were themselves dying. To characterize Konstantin's experience only as everyday feelings of loneliness and being misunderstood would miss an important point. He makes it quite clear that the problem is precisely the gap between himself (as a dying person) and the non-dying. Similarly, failing to acknowledge that the only person Judith really wants to be close to is, of all people, another dying person would neglect a crucial characteristic of her new friendship. Nor is her search for some kind of guidance while dying adequately explained as an ordinary need for security and orientation. However, by viewing Judith's and Konstantin's stories through the lens of liminal asymmetries, I can describe and analyse many of their statements and feelings without either devaluing them as mere individual moods that any non-dying person might also experience or overstating their significance as an assumed repression of the dying from the realm of the non-dying (which is not true in either case).

What I refer to here as liminal asymmetry extends beyond the fact that liminality in dying may be unaccompanied and unguided, leading to confusion, stress, and challenging situations in relations between the dying and the non-dying. That asymmetry refers ultimately to the liminal imbalances and difficulties of dying as opposed to other liminal phases marked by guidance and companionship. Other closely related facets of liminal asymmetry include the experience of hierarchy. First, simply by going through a liminal phase, dying persons gain privileged access to a mode of being that the non-dying have not yet entered. This affords the dying a certain hierarchical superiority in terms of the modes of experience they can understand from an emic point of view. Second, and at the same time, having accepted a terminal diagnosis as a reliable statement about their present and future, the dying may find themselves in a less privileged state of being than the non-dying, as they lack the full agency or status of a living person and must assume they will soon be dead and can do nothing about it. The term *liminal asymmetry* encompasses all of the ontological and capability-related hierarchies at play when the dying and the non-dying meet (including interlocutor and researcher), all of which are connected to and initiated by the opposing conditions of being or not being in a particular liminal phase.

Concluding Remarks

As I have observed in Germany and other European contexts (such as Finland), the possibility of being aware of one's state as a dying person depends on the idea that biomedical diagnoses are now relatively exact and reliable. This idea is historically and culturally quite new and became widespread only when biomedical diagnoses acquired their current meaning. It is unsurprising, then, that the liminal phase has not yet been fully unfolded to offer comprehensive guidance, initiation by the already initiated, appropriate companionship, and a concrete prospect of personal reintegration; in short, key liminal characteristics (TURNER 1967, 1974) are still missing. While institutionalized and culturally conceptualized

options for liminal guidance and communitas in dying are not (yet?) the norm, some dying persons seem to long for these features, seeking insights into the dying processes of others because the advice and companionship of the non-dying is inadequate and/or insufficient.

I have argued here that it is useful for non-dying researchers to keep these deficits of liminal guidance and communitas in mind when engaging with dying interlocutors. In so doing, we can develop a better anthropological understanding of situations that might otherwise evoke feelings of helplessness or inadequacy and fears of irritation or intrusion Acknowledging this liminal asymmetry also respects the fact that, as researchers, we can never fully provide satisfactory liminal companionship, let alone guidance, for the dying person. We can, however, show our understanding of this fact whenever we enter into close and long-term contact with someone who is terminally ill.

I have proposed to conceptualize the onto-hierarchical differences and imbalances that may arise in contacts between dying and non-dying persons as *liminal asymmetries.* In using this term, I am addressing three often interrelated dimensions that can shape and influence relationships between the dying and the non-dying. 1) The non-dying cannot access certain states of being experienced by the dying, who are not themselves prepared for the liminality of dying. 2) For some people, the desire to balance the uncertainties of liminality with companionship and guidance remains unfulfilled, rendering the liminal experience asymmetrical. This contrasts with classical Turnerian liminality, where those uncertainties and challenges are complemented by offers of guidance and companionship from people who are familiar with the particular liminal phase in question. 3) There is a crucial difference between non-dying and dying as modes of being; in the latter case, the ontological state changes as soon as the dying person acknowledges the terminal diagnosis as a reliable statement about the nature of their existence and future.

What I describe as liminal asymmetry can be observed in quite different contexts, marked by particular characteristics in each case. Researchers have described and analysed these concrete instances of onto-hierarchical asymmetries in the relationships between dying persons and professional caregivers, between the dying person and their (sometimes distant) family, and between the dying person and the ethnographer (see for example CHATTERJI 2016; ESCHENBRUCH 2007; LAWTON 2000; BECKER 2002; KRAWCZYK & RICHARDS 2021; BARRETT 2011), paying detailed attention to the specific dynamics of these contexts. Nevertheless, I contend that the more general view of these dynamics proposed here adds further value. In particular, such attempts to conceptualize the general existential differences between aware-of-dying and non-dying persons enrich theoretical efforts to understand the social meanings and dynamics of dying and death[10] by offering a decisively *anthropological* perspective on the onto-hierarchical specificities that shape relations between the terminally ill and the non-dying. This position echoes recent claims that anthropology adds nuanced complexity (SILVERMAN ET AL. 2021) to conventional readings of death-related dynamics such as grieving processes (see CORR & DOKA 2001). These conventional readings are typically rooted in particular psychological concepts that may not be designed for cross-cultural application and are unable to fully capture all that dying entails (IBID.). In contrast, my analyses of the stories of Konstantin and Judith show how a re-reading of Turner can capture certain aspects of dying that non-anthropological concepts, to my knowledge, fail to explain with similar precision.

Viewing the dynamics of dying in terms of liminal asymmetries between the dying and the non-dying also extends and revives the potential of the concept of liminality in this context as something more than a commonplace. For me at least, this also illuminates how, as researchers, we can find ourselves in situations that seem to entail two modes of participant observation at the same time: an inevitable involvement in the interlocutor's experiences and an essential inability to truly share their views and feelings.

Acknowledgements

My deep gratitude to all of the terminally ill interlocutors I was allowed to meet. Sincere thanks also to the anonymous reviewers and to Julia Rehsmann, Veronika Siegl, Molly Fitzpatrick, and Marcos Freire de Andrade Neves for their helpful suggestions and comments on earlier versions of the text. I thank Wolfgang Tress for everything. We miss you incredibly.

Notes

1 In this text, I address as '(aware-of) dying' those persons who consciously experience the prospect of fading away soon – that is, those who has been informed of a terminal illness that will lead to physical exitus in the near future and regard this information as a valid statement about their reality and future. There are fundamentally different ideas about how long dying lasts, when it begins, or how it is shaped by dying and non-dying persons (see for example STONINGTON 2020; AULINO 2019; for an overview, see MENZFELD 2018b). However, in the specific context referred to here, I define the dying phase as the period from receiving a terminal diagnosis to physical exitus.

2 Besides the UK palliative carers mentioned by BORGSTRÖM ET AL. (2020), this attitude is found among palliative and terminal carers in different regions of Europe (see for example BAUSEWEIN ET AL. 2015; KRÄNZLE ET AL. 2007). I have witnessed it many times since commencing my training in my early twenties as a volunteer in terminal/end-of-life care in Cologne and subsequently as a terminal carer. My experiences in this regard mirror those of other terminal carers I have met over the years who were trained in different European countries.

3 They do not refer to Turner or to his predecessor-in-thought VAN GENNEP (2006[1909]) but argue that modern fellowships in dying (end-of-life-care/companionship) is more likely to take the form of public self-revelation, sometimes through social networks.

4 This is the case even in institutional settings that bring dying persons together spatially; there is no conventionalized procedure to promote or enable exchange between dying persons in either hospice or palliative care units.

5 This topos has been acted upon by different groups and movements attempting to counteract the perceived repression of death and dying. For an example of counter-activism, see LOFLAND (1978); for an academic account of recent group and company attempts to re-naturalize and socially re-embed supposed repression of death and dying, see WESTENDORP & GOULD (2021).

6 As we will see, however, some dying persons seek companionship in literature and weblogs written by other dying persons.

7 This may also differ from the situation of those directly confronted with death and dying in different contexts – for example, because they live in regions where war dictates the rhythm of life, because they intend to become a suicide bomber, or because they are awaiting a death sentence. In these latter cases, factors such as the (non)existence of a subjective death wish, risk tolerance, ideas of improvement (e.g. of one's own soul or family nutritional situation) are formative. In all such cases, one's fundamental bodily capacity to continue living is threatened but is not imagined as unalterably or irrevocably absent. It is different when a person assumes that their own body itself limits their life or when an external factor or a decision of some kind is involved in limiting their life.

8 Judith's reservations certainly stemmed in part from having to take advice from people who were more educated and better-off than herself. However, as she referred explicitly to age differences and life experience, I also stress these dimensions here.

9 I would have liked to say more about her friend here. However, for their own reasons, his family did not feel comfortable with my use of most of the notes and quotes that refer to him.

10 See for example influential psychiatric-psychoanalytical and sociological classics as KÜBLER-ROSS (1973) or GLASER & STRAUSS (1965) and well-known historians like ARIÈS (1976) or recent biomedical contributions (ALBRECHT 2015; HUTTER ET AL. 2015).

References

ALBRECHT, ELISABETH 2015. Terminalphase und Tod. Der Sterbevorgang. In BAUSEWEIN, CLAUDIA; ROLLER, SUSANNE & VOLTZ, RAYMOND (eds) *Leitfaden Palliative Care: Palliativmedizin und Hospizbetreuung.* München: Urban & Fischer, 340–43.

ANDRADE NEVES, MARCOS FREIRE DE 2022. Afterlife reverberations: practices of un/naming in ethnographic research on assisted suicide. *Curare* 45, 2: 15–25.

APPLETON, JANE 2004. Ethical Issues in narrative research in palliative care. In KALITZKUS, VERA & TWOHIG, PETER (eds) *Making Sense of Health, Illness and Disease.* Amsterdam/New York: Rodopi: 259–276.

ARIÈS, PHILIPPE 1976. *Western Attitudes Toward Death from the Middle Ages to the Present.* London: Marion Boyars.
——— 1981. *The Hour of Our Death.* London: Allen Lane.

AULINO, FELICITY 2019. *Rituals of Care: Karmic Politics in an Aging Thailand.* Ithaca: Cornell University Press.

BARRETT, RON 2011. Anthropology at the end of life. In SINGER, MERRILL & ERICKSON, PAMELA (eds) *A Companion to Medical Anthropology.* Oxford: Wiley-Blackwell: 477–90.

BAUSEWEIN, CLAUDIA; ROLLER, SUSANNE & RAYMOND VOLTZ 2015. *Leitfaden Palliative Care: Palliativmedizin und Hospizbetreuung.* München: Urban & Fischer.

BECKER, ERNEST 1973. *The Denial of Death.* New York: The Free Press.

BECKER, GAY 2002. Dying away from home: quandaries of migration for elders in two ethnic groups. *Journals Of Gerontology* 57, 2: 79–95.

BEHAR, RUTH 1996. *The Vulnerable Observer. Anthropology that Breaks your Heart.* Boston: Beacon Press.

BORGSTROM, ERIKA; COHN, SIMON & DRIESSEN, ANNELIEKE 2020. "We come in as 'the nothing'": researching non-intervention in palliative care. *Medicine Anthropology Theory* 7, 2: 202–13. https://doi.org/10.17157/mat.7.2.769

CHATTERJI, ROMA 2016. The experience of death in a Dutch nursing home: on touching the Other. In DAS, VEENA &

HAN, CLARA (eds) *Living and Dying in the Contemporary World. A Compendium.* Oakland: University of California Press: 696–711.

CORR, CHARLES & KENNETH DOKA 2001. Master concepts in the field of death, dying, and bereavement: coping versus adaptive strategies. *Omega* 43, 3: 183–99.

ESCHENBRUCH, NICHOLAS 2007. *Nursing Stories – Life and Death in a German Hospice.* Oxford: Berghahn Books.

FITZPATRICK, MOLLY 2022. From 'Being There' to 'Being With': Negotiating Affect and Intimacy while doing Ethnography at the Beginning of Life. *Curare* 45, 2: 37–50.

GLASER, BARNEY & STRAUSS, ANSELM 1965. *Awareness of Dying.* Chicago: Aldine.

GIDDENS, ANTHONY 1991. *Modernity and Self-Identity.* Cambridge: Polity.

HERRNDORF, WOLFGANG 2013. *Arbeit und Struktur.* Berlin: Rowohlt.

HUTTER, NICO; STÖSSEL, ULRICH; MEFFERT, CORNELIA; KÖRNER, MIRIAM; BOZZARRO, CLAUDIA; BECKER, GERHILD & BAUMEISTER, HARALD 2015. "Good dying". Definition and current state of research. *Deutsche Medizinische Wochenschrift* 140, 17: 1296–1301.

KAUFMAN, SHARON & MORGAN, LYNN 2005. The anthropology of the beginnings and ends of life. *Annual Review of Anthropology* 34, 3: 17–41.

KAUFMAN, SHARON 2000. Senescence, decline, and the quest for a good death: contemporary dilemmas and historical antecedents. *Aging Studies* 14, 1: 1–23.

KRÄNZLE, SUSANNE; SCHMID, ULRIKE & SEEGER, CHRISTA 2007. *Palliative Care. Handbuch für Pflege und Begleitung.* Berlin/Heidelberg: Springer Medizin Verlag.

KRAWCZYK, MARIAN & RICHARDS, NAOMI 2021. A critical rejoinder to "Life's End: Ethnographic Perspectives". *Death Studies* 45, 5: 405–12. https://doi.org/10.1080/07481187.2019.1639903

KÜBLER-ROSS, ELISABETH 1973. *Interviews mit Sterbenden.* Stuttgart: Kreuz Verlag.

LAWTON, JULIA 2000. *The Dying Process: Patients' Experiences of Palliative Care.* London: Routledge. https://doi.org/10.4324/9780203130278

LEMOS DEKKER, NATASHE 2019. Standing at the doorstep: affective encounters in research on death and dying. In STODULKA, THOMAS; DINKELAKER, SAMIA & THAJIB FERDIANSYAH (eds) *Affective Dimensions of Fieldwork and Ethnography. Theory and History in the Human and Social Sciences.* Cham: Springer. https://doi.org/10.1007/978-3-030-20831-8_18
——— 2018. Moral frames for lives worth living: managing the end of life with dementia. *Death Studies* 42, 5: 322–28. https://doi.org/10.1080/07481187.2017.1396644

LOFLAND, LYN 1978. *The Craft of Dying: The Modern Face of Death.* Beverly Hills: SAGE.

LONG, SUSAN 2004. Cultural scripts for a good death in Japan and the United States: similarities and differences. *Social Science & Medicine* 58, 5: 913–28. https://doi.org/10.1016/j.socscimed.2003.10.037

MATTINGLY, CHERYL 1998. In search of the Good: narrative reasoning in clinical practice. *Medical Anthropology Quar-*

terly 12, 3: 273–297. https://doi.org/10.1525/maq.1998.12.3.273

MENZFELD, MIRA 2022. Silent questions: (not) talking about dying in the Pearl River Delta. *Medicine Anthropology Theory* 9, 2: 1–10.

——— 2021. Zum Schreien. Les émotions "troublantes" ressenties par des personnes en situation de mourir pré-exital en Allemagne. / Zum Schreien. Experiencing uncanny emotions as a pre-exitally dying person in Germany. *Anthropologie et Sociétés* 45, 1–2: 109–33. https://doi.org/10.7202/1083797ar

——— 2018a. *Anthropology of Dying*. Wiesbaden: Springer.

——— 2018b. Und manche sterben nie. Verortungen von Sterbensprozessen im interkulturellen Vergleich. In BENKEL, THORSTEN (ed) *Zwischen Leben und Tod*. Wiesbaden: Springer: 93–108.

——— 2017. When the dying do not feel tabooed: perspectives of the terminally ill in Western Germany. *Mortality* 22, 4: 308–23. https://doi.org/10.1080/13576275.2016.1270261

NASSEHI, ARMIN 2006 [2004]. Formen der Vergesellschaftung des Sterbeprozesses. In NATIONALER ETHIKRAT DER BUNDESREPUBLIK DEUTSCHLAND (ed) *Tagungsdokumentationen: Wie wir sterben/ Selbstbestimmung am Lebensende. Tagungen des Nationalen Ethikrates in Augsburg und Münster:* 81–94. https://www.ethikrat.org/fileadmin/Publikationen/Tagungsdokumentationen/Tagungen_2004_Wie_wir_sterben-Selbstbestimmung_am_Lebensende.pdf [30.6.2022].

PALGI, PHYLLIS & ABRAMOVITCH, HENRY 1984. Death: a cross-cultural perspective. *Annual Review of Anthropology* 13, 1: 385–417.

REHSMANN, JULIA & SIEGL, VERONIKA 2022. The Beginnings and Ends of Life as a Magnifying Glass for Ethnographic Research: Introduction to the Special Issue. *Curare* 45, 2: 5-14.

RIESSMAN, CATHERINE & MATTINGLY, CHERYL 2005. Introduction: Toward a context-based ethics for social research in health. *Health* 9, 4: 427–29.

SCHLINGENSIEF, CHRISTOPH 2009. *So schön wie hier kann's im Himmel gar nicht sein! Tagebuch einer Krebserkrankung*. Köln: Kiepenheuer & Witsch.

SEALE, CLIVE 2004. Media constructions of dying alone: a form of 'bad death'. *Social Science & Medicine* 58, 5: 967–74.

SILVERMAN, GILA; BAROILLER, AURÉLIEN & HEMER, SUSAN 2021. Culture and grief: ethnographic perspectives on ritual, relationships and remembering. *Death Studies* 45, 1: 1–8. https://doi.org/10.1080/07481187.2020.1851885

STONINGTON, SCOTT 2020. *The Spirit Ambulance. Choreographing the End of Life in Thailand*. Oakland: University of California Press.

THOMPSON, KIMBERLY 2007. Liminality as a description for the cancer experience. *Illness, Crisis and Loss* 15, 4: 333–51. https://doi.org/10.2190/IL.15.4.d

TURNER, VICTOR 1964. Betwixt and between: the liminal period in rites de passage. In SPIRO, MELFORD (ed) *Symposium on New Approaches to the Study of Religion*. Seattle: American Ethnological Society: 4–20.

——— 1967. *The Forest of Symbols. Aspects of Ndembu Ritual*. London: Cornell University Press.

——— 1969. *The Ritual Process. Structure and Anti-Structure*. Chicago: Aldine Publishing.

——— 1974. *Dramas, Fields and Metaphors. Symbolic Action in Human Society*. London: Cornell University Press.

VAN DER GEEST, SJAAK 2004. Dying peacefully: considering good death and bad death in Kwahu-Tafo, Ghana. *Social Science & Medicine* 58, 5: 899–911. https://doi.org/10.1016/j.socscimed.2003.10.041

VAN GENNEP, ARNOLD 2006. The rites of passage. In ROBBEN, ANTONIUS (ed) *Death, Mourning and Burial. A Cross-Cultural Reader*. Malden: Blackwell: 213–23 [orig. 1909].

WALTER, TONY 2017. *What Death Means Now. Thinking Critically about Dying and Grieving*. Bristol: Policy Press.

——— 2003. Historical and Cultural Variants on the Good Death. *BMJ* 327, 7408: 218–20.

WALTER, TONY; HOURIZI, RACHID; MONCUR, WENDY & PITSILLIDES, STACEY 2012. Does the internet change how we die and mourn? Overview and analysis. *OMEGA – Journal of Death and Dying* 64, 4: 275–302. https://doi.org/10.2190%-2FOM.64.4.a

WESTENDORP, MARISKE & GOULD, HANNAH 2021. Re-feminizing death: gender, spirituality and death care in the Anthropocene. *Religions* 12, 8: 667. https://doi.org/10.3390/rel12080667

WOODTHORPE, KATE 2011. Researching death: methodological reflections on the management of critical distance. *International Journal of Social Research Methodology* 14, 2: 99–109.

Manuscript received: 10.03.2022
Manuscript accepted: 17.10.2022

MIRA MENZFELD | Dr. phil., is a cultural and social anthropologist and works as an advanced postdoc researcher in the University Research Priority Programme 'Digital Religion(s)' at the Department of Religious Studies, University of Zurich. Her areas of specialization include the anthropology of dying, the anthropology of religion (with a focus on Islam and religious 'digitability'), and the anthropology of emotions, especially in (polygynous) couple relationships. She has conducted fieldwork with terminally ill people, European Salafis, and transmigrants in Switzerland, Finland, South China, and Germany. As a former journalist, Mira is particularly concerned with the transfer of anthropological knowledge into public contexts.

University of Zurich
Religionswissenschaftliches Seminar / UFSP Digital Religion(s)
Kantonsschulstrasse 1, 8001 Zurich, Switzerland
mira.menzfeld@uzh.ch

Uncomfortable Care

Feeling through Ways of 'Being With' as a Doula-Ethnographer

MOLLY FITZPATRICK

Abstract When doing research at the beginning and end of life, ethnographers often feel the urge to engage in the care of the people they are studying. In this paper, I reflect on my attempts to provide care as a volunteer doula, a non-medical birth support person, while conducting ethnographic fieldwork on childbirth in two midwifery clinics in Bali, Indonesia. Becoming a doula-ethnographer meant going beyond silent observation – what might be called 'being there' – to 'be with' women in labour. In this article, I explore this mode of being with, and show how it centres on witnessing, letting things happen, and not going in with an agenda. As my experiences show, caring in the mode of being with was also often uncomfortable and riddled with complex ethical considerations. In this paper, I stay with and reflect on this discomfort to show how the affective negotiations of my attempts to care for women in labour led me to crucial ethnographic insights.

Keywords childbirth – ethnography – doula – care – affect

Introduction

About a week after starting my doctoral research at a private maternity clinic in Bali, Indonesia, the midwives invited me to attend a birth. I was both excited and hesitant to accept their invitation because I was not sure what my role would be as an ethnographer during such an intimate and existential moment as childbirth. After receiving the birthing woman and her husband's approval, I decided to stand in the corner of the room and try not to get in anyone's way. As the daughter of a midwife, I had been present at a birth before. Despite this familiarity, the intensity of what I witnessed overwhelmed me. I was in awe of the raw and real strength of the woman in labour, and a tear rolled down my cheek when I heard the baby let out its first cry. However, my unclear position made me feel uncomfortable – taking notes in the corner felt disconnected and strange during such an emotional and intense event.

Over the course of my fieldwork, I gradually moved out of the corner of the birthing room. After completing a course at a second midwifery clinic on the island, I became more involved in the care of women during labour by volunteering as a doula, a non-medical birth support person.

In this paper, I reflect on this journey and my experiences of combining research with the provision of care as what I call a doula-ethnographer. Engaging actively in the care of interlocutors is quite a common practice in medical anthropology. Examples are ANGELA GARCIA (2010), who worked the graveyard shift as a detoxification attendant at the heroin detoxification clinic she was researching in New Mexico, and LISA STEVENSON (2014), who volunteered at a suicide hotline when studying youth suicide in Inuit communities in the Canadian Arctic. Furthermore, I am not the first anthropologist to train as a doula in order to gain access to and do research on childbirth (FORD 2020; SCHIAVENATO 2020; STRONG 2020). However, such a double role requires extensive reflection and ethical consideration. What challenges might we face as caring ethnographers? What does it mean to engage in care during research in such settings and, in particular, at the beginning of life?

Approaching those we study with care has been described as a key feminist research value (ELLINGSON 1998; REINHARZ 1993). However, RACHELLE CHADWICK (2021: 557) argues that the values of empathy and care can gloss over the hierarchies and power imbalances between researchers and interlocutors, thereby flattening and reinforcing differences between women (CHADWICK 2021: 559, see also HEMMINGS 2012: 152). Drawing on her experiences conducting research on childbirth in South Africa, she contrasts care as a research method with what she calls "staying with discomfort" (CHADWICK 2021: 559). As she argues, "acknowledging, and staying with, messy ambivalences, sticky discomforts, falterings, disconnections, epistemic uncertainty and the intense feelings often evoked in/through research interactions is critical to efforts to develop ethical and accountable feminist research" (CHADWICK 2021: 559). I agree with the need to stay with discomfort, and in this article I do not shy away from the stickiness, messiness, and ambivalence of research – both in the role of a silent observer and as a doula-ethnographer. However, I also wish to challenge Chadwick's opposition between care and empathy on the one hand, and discomfort and ambivalence on the other. Instead, I argue, that engaging in care is often in and of itself messy, and attempts to care do not necessarily mean that interactions become smooth and devoid of discomfort or awkwardness.

In this paper, I show how doula work can provide an avenue for going beyond mere observation – or 'being there' – towards 'being with', a mode of engagement that is more in line with the aims of ethnography. As my experiences reveal, though, the ways in which I tried to be with as a doula-ethnographer were not straightforward nor easy. In order to highlight its inherent stickiness, to foreground the discomfort associated with it, and to point to the power asymmetries that underlie it, I refer to my care as a doula-ethnographer as uncomfortable care. Similar to EMILY YATES-DOERR's concept of "antihero care" (2020), my focus on uncomfortable care aims to embrace the partiality and vulnerability of ethnographic fieldwork. Instead of aiming for a complete and holistic picture of the field, which is never truly obtainable, YATES-DOERR (2020: 241) argues that we should instead depart from a notion of interdependence and care, thereby foregrounding the importance of making good connections. As I will show, engaging in uncomfortable care as doula-ethnographer led to

key research insights not because it gave me better research access or meant that I was present in more situations (more 'theres'). Rather, it was through the intimate and trusting relationships I built with the people I accompanied and my affective engagements with them that my research (and I myself as a person) benefited the most.

Context and Positionality

I travelled to Bali to study two birthing clinics, each founded by an American midwife and staffed by Indonesian midwives. The founders of these clinics were strongly influenced by the natural childbirth movement, which emerged in Europe and North America in the 1960s and 1970s as a movement against the medicalisation of birth (DAVISS 2001: 70). Based on the idea that a woman's body is made for childbirth, proponents of this movement argued that the birthing process is not eased through but rather disrupted by medical interventions. Proponents of natural birth criticize the language of risk that is central to modern obstetrics, and they argue that birth should not be seen as an illness to be cured with technology but rather as a natural process that is interrupted when it is moved to the hospital (DAVIS FLOYD 1994). Therefore, they advocate for home birth or birth in non-medical clinics and promote the idea of natural pain relief using water, breathing techniques, movement, and massage. Drawing on a range of literature on natural birth and the careful negotiation and construction it requires (ANNANDALE 1988; MACDONALD 2006, 2007; PASVEER & AKRICH 2001; SKEIDE 2020), the main focus of my research was to understand how these clinics drew on the natural birth movement in discourse and practice within the Indonesian context.

On the one hand, the discourse of natural childbirth posits birth in countries such as Indonesia as more "authentic", "traditional", and "close to nature" (MACDONALD 2007: 56); on the other hand, rising C-section rates and the general medicalisation and hospitalisation of healthcare in these countries are seen as threats to women's autonomy and their self-determination regarding birth experiences. This means that such countries are attractive places for natural birthing clinics, which both aim to address the medicalisation of birth and draw on the 'naturalness' associated with these places. Bali is a prime example of this – an island that has long held a position in the Western imagination as "the 'enchanted isle', 'the last paradise', one of the world's great romantic dreams" (VICKERS 1989: 1). In recent decades, Bali has become a mecca for all things wellness, including yoga, alternative healing therapies, and clean eating. A well-established community of foreigners lives on the island, many of whom work in the wellness sector themselves, amongst whom the clinics were a popular place for perinatal care. There were also Indonesian women who travelled from other islands to give birth in these clinics and the occasional foreigner who travelled from abroad to Bali specifically to give birth.

The clinics biggest client group and main focus, however, were Indonesian women who lived in the area of the clinics, and were either Balinese or migrants from other Indonesian islands. With this main demographic of local working-class people in mind, the services at the clinics are made affordable through the support of aid organisations and local charities. At the smaller of the two clinics, women pay a small fee for services comparable to the prices at government clinics, while at the larger clinic, Indonesian women can access services on a pay-as-you-can basis. Foreigners who come to this clinic, however, are asked to pay around 1000 US dollars for their births, which is framed as a donation in order to keep the clinic running and free for locals.[1]

Before I embarked on my research, I learnt Indonesian for six months. By the time I was in the field, I was able to both conduct interviews and support women during birth in Indonesian. My research spanned several visits to Bali and Java for a total of nine months. Over this period, I attended fourteen births, the first six as an observer and the following eight as a volunteer doula. Apart from one woman from Switzerland and one woman from the US, all the women I saw give birth were Indonesian. These women were either from working-class or lower middle-class backgrounds, and while the low prices often played a role in their considerations for choosing the clinics, many of them were motivated by a wish to give birth vaginally and without medical interventions. Besides the midwives and the couple,

I was not the only person present during these births. Almost all couples brought along several family members and sometimes friends, and there were often quite a few people walking in and out of the birthing room. When chatting with family members, I was often told that, in the village, it was an usual practice for the whole community to wait outside a woman's house when she was in labour. In this sense, labour and birth are deeply social events in Indonesia.

During the first few births I observed, I wondered whether my status as a young white woman meant that I was invited into the birthing room more easily and that my presence was less questioned. As the clinics had previously hosted foreign midwifery students observing births as part of an internship abroad, I seemed to slot rather seamlessly into that role. A common question I was asked was when I would finish my studies as a midwife. Although I made an effort of repeating that I was doing a PhD in Cultural Anthropology, not being a midwifery student made my role rather ambiguous. I did not fit into any of the existing roles in the clinic, as is often the case with ethnography in clinics and hospitals (WIND 2008).

My positionality as a young white woman also deserves further reflection, as the broader power imbalances and hierarchies that underlie my research contributed to my discomfort when observing births. I am a Dutch citizen (although I live in Switzerland and work for a Swiss university, which came with its own connotations of wealth and privilege) and was conducting research in a former Dutch colony. Making notes and attempting to remain removed from the interactions unfolding in front of me seemed to contribute to my status as supposedly objective outsider, a historically problematic status when it comes to colonialism and anthropology's role therein. In this way, I felt that my research, and, in particular, the way in which I stood in the corner of the birthing room taking notes, could be seen through the lens of ongoing asymmetrical knowledge production between former coloniser and colony.

I thus spent the first part of my research standing awkwardly in the corner, unsure of my role and aware of my (white) privilege, repeating that I was an anthropologist to people who were too busy to care, all the while wondering how to understand the bodily and affective processes of care that were unfolding in front of me.

Beyond Being There

In the introduction to this special issue, JULIA REHSMANN & VERONIKA SIEGL (2022) draw on a rich array of literature to illustrate the importance of studying processes of giving birth and dying. As their discussion shows, studying the beginning and end of life not only provides crucial insights into the very fundamentals of what it means to be human, but also raises many methodological questions, in particular regarding how to approach such experiences ethnographically. As MIRA MENZFELD (this issue) argues in her contribution, understanding such non-delegable experiences as birthing and dying from an emic perspective is impossible. Researchers are unlikely to be dying themselves, and even if they have given birth, the acutely bodily experience of being in labour is different for everyone. Further, the beginning and end of life concern liminal and existential phases that often include intense pain and altered perception (REHSMANN & SIEGL, this issue). This makes participant observation during such processes difficult, as busy medical staff often does not have time to interact, and the people experiencing labour and birth or dying are often unable to do so. The role of the ethnographer becomes unclear and potentially cumbersome for the research participants, as I experienced during the first births I observed.

Simply observing silently and taking notes when your research participants are going through intense pain and emotions can thus feel inappropriate and uncomfortable. In her book of personal essays, *The Vulnerable Observer* (1996), RUTH BEHAR constructs perhaps one of the most beautifully written critiques of observation without emotional engagement. As she asserts, "nothing is stranger than the business of humans observing other humans in order to write about them" (BEHAR 1996: 5). For her, this strangeness is mainly due to the fact that researchers are expected to conceal their own emotions when observing. This seems impossible to Behar, as emotions are key to anthropology. For her, anthropology is about

loss, mourning, the longing for memory, the desire to enter into the world around you and having no idea how to do it, the fear of observing too coldly or too distractedly or too raggedly, the rage of cowardice, [...] a sense of utter uselessness of writing anything and yet the burning desire to write something (BEHAR 1996: 3)

This poignant description places the affective negotiations of ethnography and writing front and centre, revealing that pure observation perpetuates the myth that we can filter out our own emotions while doing research.

BEHAR's critique of only 'being there' highlights the need to develop an affective methodology, something that has long been key to a feminist approach to ethnography (THAJIB ET AL. 2019: 15; STOLLER 2019). For some authors, emotions play a role mainly in creating rapport and negotiating different situations during fieldwork (BERGMAN BLIX & WETTERGREN 2015; CAROLL 2012; DICKSON-SWIFT ET AL. 2009; HOLMES 2010). Other authors push further and argue that affects should play a central role not only in our methodological approach but also in our analysis. Similar to CHADWICK, JULIA REHSMANN (2019: 198) shows how taking discomfort seriously, as a starting point for emotional reflexivity, can greatly enrich the ethnographic endeavour of understanding the human condition. For sensitive topics and intimate, emotionally-charged situations, such as birth and death, an affective methodology is even more crucial (DICKSON-SWIFT ET AL. 2009; CHADWICK 2021; OAKLEY 1981; SAMPSON ET AL. 2008). Affect is often elusive and difficult to see as it moves between (human and non-human) bodies, is attached to spaces and objects, and is subjectively felt (KNUDSEN & STAGE 2015: 5). This links back to the need to go beyond 'being there' towards bodily engagement. One way to engage bodily could be to take an active role in caring for people who are giving birth or dying.

The experiences of other ethnographers who study the beginning and end of life show how it can also become unethical *not* to engage. During her fieldwork in a public maternity ward in Tanzania, ADRIENNE STRONG (2020) witnessed many infant and maternal deaths, thereby conducting fieldwork at both the beginning and end of life simultaneously. While she had not intended to deliver babies, the dire situation of scarcity she encountered at the hospital led her to state that "simply scribbling away in my little black notebook had become untenable" (STRONG 2020: 18). After receiving a short training, she attended women who would otherwise have given birth alone, often on the floor of the delivery room or in the corridor of the ward because there were not enough beds (STRONG 2020: 18). She stresses, "to not engage in the ways in which I was invited to would have been a form of ethical violation when I was there and capable of doing so" (STRONG 2020: 19). STRONG's experiences show the strong urge ethnographers might feel to contribute, in some way, to the care of interlocutors in pain. However, Strong's experiences of fieldwork are very different to mine. The clinics in Bali were not places of scarcity and abandonment, and no babies or mothers died in their birthing rooms. As for me, I did not deliver any babies. Instead, half-way through my fieldwork, I trained as a doula – a non-medical birth support person.

Becoming a Doula

After several months of research and attending several births as an observer in the smaller of the two clinics, I decided to extend my research to a second, larger natural birth clinic on the island. The midwife who started this clinic knew that I had observed births and said that I could also be present at births in her clinic. However, she wanted me to volunteer as a doula rather than to stand in the corner taking notes. She suggested I join the yearly doula retreat that she organised together with a well-known American doula. I took her up on this suggestion because I was eager to step out of the corner of the birthing room. I was aware that that volunteering as a doula, as a way to conduct research on birth, would come with its own ethical considerations. At the same time, I thought that if I was there during births, I might as well try to contribute something through my presence.

The doula retreat was two weeks and took place in Bali. It was attended by women from all over the world – including the US, Australia, Germany, France, and South Africa. In addition, three Indonesian women participated with

a scholarship offered by the clinic. This scholarship was the only way in which it was feasible for these Indonesian women to join the course, as attendance cost upwards of 2000 dollars (including food and lodgings). The women who joined the course were mostly from white, middle-class backgrounds. While some had given birth several times and attended dozens of births, others did not have children of their own and had never been present at a birth. What was striking was that almost all of the women were practicing a profession that they wanted to combine with being doula, such as teaching (prenatal) yoga, massage therapy, or practicing traditional Chinese medicine. Doula work was thus situated within a larger economy of wellness and alternative medicine and was seen by most women as an additional skill that they wanted to add to their repertoire. In and of itself, this course was a fascinating space for understanding the role that Bali plays within the global natural childbirth movement, of which doulas are often a part. These women saw Bali as both a centre for wellness and alternative medicine and a place that is implicitly associated with 'the natural', and therefore as the ideal place to learn how to be a doula.

The word "doula" comes from ancient Greek and means "a woman who serves". The term was first used in its current meaning in 1969 by the American anthropologist Dana Raphael – a protégée of Margaret Mead. A doula is someone who provides continuous physical, emotional, and informational support to a woman and her partner before, during, and just after birth. The fact that doulas have no medical responsibility, nor familial relationship to the birthing woman, is crucial to their role, as this means that they can provide constant support while maintaining some distance and without having to make difficult decisions. Doulas have become quite popular in the United States, where they work in both hospital and home birth settings, and their popularity in Europe is now steadily increasing (FORD 2020; MARXER 2022; NIEUWSUUR 2020). In Indonesia, there are only a handful of women practicing under this term, most of them located in Jakarta.[2] However, traditional birth attendants, or *dukun bayi*, have been providing similar support before and after birth for centuries, and have occasionally fulfilled a similar role during birth alongside a government midwife, or *bidan* (AM-BARETNANI 2012; NEWLAND 2002; NIEHOF 2014).

A broad range of research has been conducted on the benefits of doulas during birth, which shows that, amongst other outcomes, labours attended by doulas are generally shorter and with fewer complications (BOHREN ET AL. 2017; GRUBER ET AL. 2013; KOZHIMANNIL ET AL. 2016). However, in the media, doulas have sometimes been pitted against midwives, and the necessity of their role has been questioned (FITZPATRICK 2020; HOFMAN ET AL. 2020; NIEUWSUUR 2020). Furthermore, there has been discussion about the professionalisation of doulas and whether they should be regulated (MEYERSON 2019). The doulas I know mostly prefer not to be regulated as they feel this gives them more freedom to practice as they wish. However, this raises the question of what the role of the doula entails and where the boundaries of their scope of practice and responsibilities lie. In the doula course, we practiced different massage techniques, learnt how to help women move into different positions that improve foetal positioning, and had sessions on birth trauma, breastfeeding, and belly binding. However, what doulas actually do during birth varies and often they do not do very much at all.

Instead, the support a doula provides is often about being a constant and reassuring presence. Indeed, there is a common joke amongst doulas that they should call themselves 'belas', as their role is more about 'be'-ing (with) rather than 'do'-ing. You cannot give birth for someone, and while 'natural' pain relief, such as massage and water, can be beneficial for certain women in labour, it is not possible to take pain away completely without medical interventions. Furthermore, some women do not like to be touched at all, and longer verbal exchanges are often not possible due to the hormonally induced altered state women enter during labour. So in most cases, being a doula simply means 'being with' women and their partners throughout the journey of birth.

In this sense, and as I will show, it does not differ much from accompanying people as an ethnographer. For me, however, becoming a doula did mean taking on a certain responsibility for the women and partners who allowed me to accompany them. Once I had committed to being someone's doula, I felt a responsibility to contribute something to the woman's birth experience through my presence. This feeling of responsibility sometimes came into conflict with my role as a researcher. Before I get into those tensions, however, I will first elaborate on the idea of being with, a mode of care often employed in both midwifery and palliative care.

Ways of Being With

The idea of being with appears in many popular and academic writings on midwifery and is often seen as a characteristic of midwifery care that distinguishes it from obstetric care (BRADFIELD ET AL. 2018; HUNTER 2002; DICKSON 1996; KAUFMAN 1993). Indeed, the very term 'midwife' means 'with woman', a fact often mentioned when describing the woman-led approach that is typical of midwifery (HUNTER 2002: 651). ANNE-KATRIN SKEIDE argues that the mode of being with is enacted in midwifery through witnessing, which she defines as "embodied interrelatedness in a particular environment" (2018: 192). SKEIDE (2018: 195) invokes the stereotype of the knitting midwife to illustrate how the midwife employs witnessing as active-passive care: she seems to just sit and knit without doing much, but actually, she is watching, listening, and feeling. The passive-active care provided by the knitting midwife enables women to trust their own bodies during birth, as the fact that she sits silently and observes reassures women that what they are going through is normal and does not require action (SKEIDE 2018).

This is something I also often saw in Bali. The midwives remained quite passive during early labour, often not staying in the birthing room and only checking in every hour or so. As Sandra, the founder of one of the two clinics, described it: "For me, the best birth means a natural – I don't know if 'untouched' is a better word – birth. You know, just quietly observing. Letting it happen." Sandra describes the key to midwifery care in these clinics as a *not doing* rather than a *doing*. The care of the midwife becomes implicated in the construction of a 'natural' birth.[3] However, quietly observing and letting birth happen was only one aspect of care in these in clinics – both midwives and birthing women repeatedly stressed that care "from the heart" (*dengan hati*) was also key to creating a natural birth. Caring for women from the heart required emotional labour from the midwives, as it meant being warm and loving but also attending to the birthing women's emotions. Being with women as a midwife in these clinics thus had both a passive (letting birth happen) and active (emotional labour) element.

When it comes to care at the end of life, the importance of witnessing people's suffering and being with people who are dying is often described as the key to good palliative care (DRIESSEN ET AL. 2021). As ANNELIEKE DRIESSEN ET AL. found during research with palliative carers in the UK, being with is established not by saying or doing something, but "through not saying something or entering the conversation with an agenda, and not doing something" (DRIESSEN ET AL. 2021: 17). In his contribution to this issue, MARCOS ANDRADE NEVES (2022) gives a beautiful description of how being with someone who is dying might look like in practice. Therein, the intimate bond he has with his dying friend and interlocutor Margot is enacted through his mode of being with as he holds her hand during her last breaths. In LISA STEVENSON's work on the suicide epidemic amongst Inuit youth, her understanding of care evokes very similar notions as what DRIESSEN ET AL. and ANDRADE NEVES refer to as being with. Writing against ANNEMARIE MOL and her colleagues' notion of care as an always active doing – what they call 'tinkering' (MOL ET AL. 2010) – STEVENSON argues that care can also consist of waiting and "allowing situations – and people's lives – to unfold" (STEVENSON 2014: 177).

Witnessing, letting things happen, allowing situations to unfold, and not going in with an agenda thus constitute key characteristics of being with. This mode of care seems to be particularly common to care at the beginning and end of life, perhaps because of the existential nature and singularity of these experiences (MENZFELD, this issue; REHSMANN & SIEGL, this issue). Yet, while medical professionals, like midwives, bear a significant medical responsibility and therefore have to put down their proverbial knitting and act when necessary, doulas are not allowed or trained to provide medical care or make any medical decisions. For doulas, being with is the

main gift they have to offer. For this reason, it is even more important that doulas do not have an agenda and are not guided by their own expectations of a good birth. In the doula course, we were repeatedly told that we should not speak for the birthing person but rather learn how to amplify their voice. Therein, witnessing in the sense of listening to the others' hopes and fears and acknowledging them without jumping into action is essential to doula care.

The idea of witnessing also connects doula work with ethnography. Before leaving for her ethnographic fieldwork in Tanzania, STRONG (2020) had also trained as a doula. As she writes, her main goal in training as a doula was to serve as a witness to the woman's labour, whether it was a good or a bad experience. She argues that "witnessing is often the most valuable tool a doula has to offer and is not terribly different from the similar gift an adept ethnographer can provide through interviews and presence" (STRONG 2020: 18). In return for being welcomed into their interlocutors' lives, good ethnographers can give their interlocutors the 'gift' of witnessing: they make participation in their research worthwhile by listening to interlocutors' stories with empathy and trying to truly understand their experiences. In this sense, being with is both a mode of caring and a mode of exploration and engagement that ethnographers employ in the field.

In my experience, I found that the role of the doula both complements and extends the role of the ethnographer. While both are interested in accompanying someone on their journey and witnessing their experience, being a doula extends the intention of the feminist ethnographer to care for and about the people she researches and makes that care more tangible and physical. Whereas the hands of the ethnographer are mostly scribbling notes, the hands of the doula reach out to squeeze hands, rest on shoulders, and press on lower backs. As a doula, I was almost constantly in either physical contact with birthing women or maintaining eye contact with them throughout the many hours of labour (see also SCHIAVENATO 2020). This physicality and bodily engagement, the active element of the passive-active care of being with, made me aware of different things than when I was standing in the corner taking notes. However, the responsibility I felt to contribute something to the birthing experience of the women I accompanied also led to challenging situations, as I will now show.

A Balancing Act

I met Selena, a 37-year-old woman from the French speaking part of Switzerland, during a prenatal yoga class at one of the two clinics. She explained that she had come to Bali to give birth because of her complicated relationship with the baby's father, who did not want to be involved in the child's life. To escape the situation, she had decided to fly to Bali – which she called "the land of my heart" – to give birth. She had heard about the clinic during a previous trip to the island and dreamt of having a natural birth. Selena was very happy when I offered to volunteer as a doula during her labour. Though her friend from Switzerland, Emilie, would also be with her, she wanted all the support she could get.

When Selena's labour started, one of the first things she asked me was "am I almost there?" Unfortunately, her cervix was only 1 cm dilated, with still 9 cm to go. After twelve hours of labour with no progress, Selena requested to go to hospital so she could get an epidural for the pain. Emilie and I accompanied Selena and, together with two clinic midwives who were there to facilitate the transfer, we all piled into the small clinic ambulance. Upon arrival at the hospital, the clinic midwives left and the hospital midwives took over. Selena told me later that she found the hospital midwives brisk and unfriendly, and that the vaginal check one of them conducted was extremely painful. The midwife conducting the check refused to speak directly to Selena and instead told me in Indonesian that Selena's cervical dilation was still only 2 cm.[4]

After about an hour, when Emilie had shortly left the room to get some food, an obstetrician finally arrived. Despite her perfect English, she too turned her attention to me and explained that it was against their protocol to give an epidural before 5 cm dilation. I asked what other options there were for pain management and the doctor just shrugged and said, "All we can do is a C-section". I looked over to Selena, who looked up at me with pain and despair in her eyes. When I looked back at the doctor, I realised that they

both expected me to decide what to do. However, as both a doula and an ethnographer, I was neither willing nor able to make such a decision for Selena. Out of sheer desperation, the only thing I could think of was to leave the room. I excused myself to go to the toilet as I felt the tears welling up inside me. After quickly pulling myself together, I returned to the delivery room, where, fortunately, the doctor had decided to do another vaginal exam and found that Selena's cervical dilation had progressed to 6 cm.[5] With an obvious sigh of relief, Selena exclaimed that with a dilation of 6 cm, she could make it to 10 cm without pain medication. A little over three hours later, she pushed out a healthy baby girl.

Supporting women through such a life-changing yet uncertain and volatile process as a doula, I was taught to not let my own emotions or expectations play a role in the care I provided. Yet, what I experienced moved me emotionally. Trying to care for Selena and to advocate for her care with the hospital midwives and obstetrician was so frustrating and overwhelming that I could no longer hold back my tears – although I made sure to hide them from Selena, who needed me to be a calm and reassuring presence. When I think about how Selena went from utter desperation to being convinced once again that she would be able to give birth without pain medication, it still fills me with awe and admiration. Furthermore, my own frustration in trying to care for Selena helped me to understand better how much perseverance it must have taken for her to keep going. Though I could never truly understand how Selena must have felt, I was better able to grasp the complex exchange between Selena and the doctor because I was a part of it.

My own feelings of frustration and despair thus made me aware of the way women can be treated in the hospital when they are transferred from one of the midwifery clinics. As women in Indonesia told me repeatedly, care in the hospital was a lot less affective, responsive, and personalised than in the midwifery clinics I studied. Based on this experience, I had to agree with them. Feeling my way through the care in the hospital also helped me to understand how much the births in the clinics are overshadowed by a potential transfer. A transfer breaks the midwives' moral promise to care for women and negates the natural childbirth movement's ideal that all women can and should give birth without medical intervention. For this reason, birthing women, birth partners, and midwives worked hard to avoid a transfer. I referred to this as co-anticipative care work in my dissertation to illustrate the affective, future oriented, and collaborative nature of such negotiations (FITZPATRICK 2022).

Accompanying Selena in the hospital was by far the most challenging situation I faced as a doula-ethnographer. It illustrates how taking on the role of a doula-ethnographer can be a balancing act between passive and active care, between doing nothing and doing something, between witnessing and interfering. While in many instances I managed this balancing act successfully, in this moment it became too much for me. Being with women as a doula means being a continuous presence and not leaving a woman's side until after her child is born. Being with as an ethnographer also relies on continuity and physical presence, and I missed a crucial bit of observation during this birth when the obstetrician conducted an additional vaginal check. However, in that moment, staying within the boundaries of my role and not making or contributing to any medical decisions was more important to my mode of being with as a doula-ethnographer than physical presence. In this instance, and rather paradoxically, being with meant for me not being there at all.

Uncomfortable Care

As CHADWICK (2021: 557) argued, the affects circulating in research encounters, such as feelings of frustration, desperation, and discomfort, should be understood as "the products of intertwining relational, material, embodied, discursive, intersubjective and sociomaterial dynamics". These affects are crucial for understanding, interpreting, and representing the research field, as they can turn us "on" and "off" to particular lines of thinking (CHADWICK 2021: 557). As a doula-ethnographer I shared not only in the frustration and desperation when labour became complicated or took much longer than expected, but also in the joy and elation when babies finally made their appearance after hours and hours of their mother's hard work. Being present at such

a crucial and intimate moment in someone's life often meant that I created strong intimate bonds with the people I accompanied during birth. Despite the relationships it facilitated, however, being with as a doula-ethnographer did not smooth over the feelings of discomfort I described at the beginning of this paper. The underlying power asymmetries did not disappear just because I was no longer simply observing but was now engaging in care. If anything, my affective engagements made it even more pertinent to reflect on the power dynamics and ethics of my relationships and interactions in the field.

Selena and I grew close during the weeks that followed her birth, and she came to visit me in Zurich after my fieldwork ended.[6] I also stayed in contact with many of the other women I supported, and I visited them in their homes across the island. My relationships with people in the field thereby changed and evolved with time, as did the ethics of these relationships. Before leaving for Bali, I obtained ethical approval for my research from the medical faculty at Udayana University (this was required for my research visa), and I printed out informed consent forms, which I had my interlocutors sign when I first asked them to be part of my research. But as my role in the field and my relationship with interlocutors evolved and changed, so did the ethical considerations of my research. This necessitated a relational approach to ethics (ELLIS 2007; HALSE & HONEY 2005; CANELLA & LINCOLN 2007), meaning that I had to consider repeatedly what the ethical repercussions of my attempts to provide care as an ethnographer were. Let me give some examples of how my interactions with people changed when I became a doula-ethnographer.

First of all, being a doula changed the way in which I moved through the space of clinic. I spent many more hours continuously in the clinic, walked in and out of rooms quickly and with purpose, and ate meals at the table just in front of the kitchen with the midwives and other staff. This meant that, even more than before, people assumed that I had medical knowledge and expertise, and I was associated strongly with the clinics. It was common for women and their partners to walk up to me to ask (medical) questions. On several occasions, couples asked me to second guess the midwives when they had been referred to the hospital due to a pre-existing condition or indication that came up during pregnancy. These couples saw me as representing the values of the natural birth discourse that had attracted them to the clinic.[7] Being put in this situation by couples made me feel uncomfortable, and I always tried to deflect such questions and make sure that the couples understood that I did not have any medical expertise or authority.

Secondly, as a doula-ethnographer, I had to negotiate with many different actors and the power dynamics of these interactions were sometimes quite complex. This is illustrated by my experience supporting Cindy, a woman originally from West Papua who I met and interviewed while she waited for a prenatal check-up. When she went into labour several weeks later, she called me and asked if I could come to the clinic to support her as a doula. When I arrived, however, her mother, who was also there for support, questioned the fact that I was supporting women in labour while I had not given birth myself. She then asked to see a doctor, and when I told her there were no doctors on staff, she became angry with me and stormed out the room. While my interactions with Cindy's mother made me feel uneasy and inadequate, I stayed and supported Cindy because I thought that she wanted me there.

Such complicated and uncomfortable power dynamics are compounded during childbirth due to its existential, emotional, and intimate nature. Women who are in labour often find it difficult to talk or answer questions, and this meant that I sometimes had to assume what they wanted in order to care for them. For example, I accompanied a woman from Sumbawa named Bayu who had come to the clinic with her Australian husband because they both wanted their child to be born naturally, without medical interventions. Throughout the harder parts of her labour, however, Bayu begged me and her husband for pain medication, repeating the phrase "help me" over and over again. As I could see that she was progressing and that full dilation was imminent, I decided to gently remind her that she had chosen this clinic for a reason and that she was strong and capable of giving birth without pain medication. While Bayu later told me that she appreciated my encouraging words, as an ethnographer whose aim was to deconstruct discourses of nat-

ural birth, I felt uncomfortable reproducing and contributing to them instead.

As my experiences accompanying women like Selena, Cindy, and Bayu show, it was never possible to fully comprehend the effects that my engagements as a doula-ethnographer had, and whether I made the right decisions in my attempts at care. Due to the responsibility I felt and was perceived to have for the care of women in labour when I became a doula, I sometimes came to represent or reproduce the structures and discourses I was aiming to study. In this way, caring for women during the emotional and existential process of labour and birth was unavoidably riddled with complex ethical considerations and uncomfortable convergences. The act of care itself was thereby neither a way to smooth over unequal or awkward relations nor a way to make discomfort go away. Rather, while acknowledging and embracing the partiality and vulnerability of this mode of research, engaging in uncomfortable care helped me to better understand the complex and intricate webs of affect and care that were spun in the birthing room and beyond.

Conclusion

Being with is a mode of engagement that is central to both the way in which I cared for women as a doula and the way I related to my interlocutors as an ethnographer. Despite this commonality, I found that being with as a doula-ethnographer was often uncomfortable, difficult, and messy, and it brought up many ethical questions as my role evolved over time. This underlines that, as researchers, our engagement with ethics should not cease as soon as we have obtained ethical approval or after our informed consent forms have been signed – it should be an ongoing engagement without end. Following CHADWICK (2021), part of my commitment to an ethical and accountable feminist research practice has been to acknowledge and reflect on my feelings of discomfort in the field and the power asymmetries that underlie them. Therein, the commitment to care need not be at odds with the aim of staying with discomfort and acknowledging the stickiness of unequal relationships in the field. Instead, I argue that uncomfortable care can be a way through which to create and sustain intimate and affective relationships with people across such differences.

My experiences reveal an underlying tension when it comes to the affective dimension of being with as a doula-ethnographer. As I was taught in the doula course, I always tried to bracket my own emotions when being with women as a doula. In a paradoxical way, however, this forced me to recognise my feelings and deal with them, so as not to let them take up space in my care. Feelings, such as frustration and despair but also joy and elation, welled up inside me as I negotiated with different actors. I grappled with these emotions by writing about them in my journal and field notes and reflecting on them extensively. In the end, these reflections pointed me to the central role of affect in the natural birth movement in Indonesia, leading to key insights for my research. As I balanced active and passive care, witnessing and interfering, I was able to see how natural birth in this context relied on a balancing act from the midwives between letting birth happen and caring from the heart.

Another balancing act for me was between deconstructing and representing/reproducing the discourse I was aiming to study. There too, embodying the discourse through my engagements as a doula-ethnographer showed me how it is enacted in practice in the clinic and beyond. The bodily engagement of being with women in labour, including the sometimes uncomfortable negotiations this active-passive care required, thus became a crucial heuristic for understanding the way in which natural birth was perceived and practiced in this context.

Notes

1 During the time of my research, around four or five women gave birth in the smaller clinic on a weekly basis. At the larger clinic, there were ten or more births a week. Both clinics also attracted dozens of women a week for prenatal check-ups, and the larger of the two clinics also offered free prenatal yoga classes. It also had a general practitioner and traditional Chinese medicine practitioner on staff, who also treated (Indonesian) patients who did not come for perinatal care for free.
2 I got this information from a small group of doulas I met in Jakarta, when I visited a doula I had met at the course and stayed with her for a week.
3 I use quotation marks around the word natural here to stress that, while supposedly natural and based on

the innate capabilities of women's bodies, 'natural birth' does not just happen by itself. As other ethnographers have also shown, constituting birth as natural requires rhetorical work (MACDONALD 2007: 6), bodily negotiation (SKEIDE 2020), and technological mediation (PASVEER AND AKRICH 2001).
4 There was quite a mix of different languages spoken in the hospital. Selena only spoke a few words of Indonesian, while both Emilie and I were fluent enough to conduct conversations with the hospital midwives. While I communicated with Selena and Emilie in English, the midwives only spoke a little English. Emilie and Selena communicated with each other in French. Although I can understand some French, I cannot speak it.
5 Either the hospital midwife who had examined Selena earlier had been wrong about her cervical dilation, or the dilation had progressed extremely quickly in the last hour. It could also be that because Selena found the vaginal examination that the midwife had performed rather painful, she had contracted her muscles, making it difficult to examine her accurately.
6 Our socio-economic circumstances were quite similar, as we both lived in Switzerland and have stable jobs (Selena works as a special needs teacher in a school) with average incomes for Swiss standards. This and the fact that we were both foreigners in Bali surely facilitated our relationship. However, the similarities between us end there. Selena is almost ten years older than me and comes from an immigrant, working-class background. While my parents are also immigrants, they are white and middle-class. Our communication was also not always smooth, as Selena is fluent in French and Spanish (two languages I do not speak), but often had trouble expressing herself in English. This did not matter so much when it came to supporting her during birth and spending time with her and her newborn Maya, but when I tried to interview her more formally about her birth experience, I ended up asking her to talk in French and later had the recorded interview transcribed and translated.
7 While I do not know for sure, this might also be because of my appearance as a young white woman and the fact that the natural birth movement has been imported in its current form from Western Europe and the US to Indonesia – meaning that it was possible that the couples associated me implicitly with this discourse and its approach to birth because I am European and white.

References

AMBARETNANI, PRIHATINI 2012. *Paraji and Bidan in Rancaekek: Integrated Medicine for Advanced Partnerships among Traditional Birth Attendants and Community Midwives in the Sunda Region of West Java, Indonesia*. PhD Dissertation: Leiden University.

ANDRADE NEVES, MARCOS 2022. Afterlife Reverberations: Practices of Un/naming in Ethnographic Research on Assisted Suicide. *Curare* 45, 2: 15–25.

ANNANDALE, ELLEN 1988. How Midwives Accomplish Natural Birth: Managing Risk and Balancing Expectations. *Social Problems* 35, 2: 95–110.

APPIAH, KWAME ANTHONY 2020. The Case for Capitalizing the *B* in Black. *The Atlantic*. https://www.theatlantic.com/ideas/archive/2020/06/time-to-capitalize-blackand-white/613159/ [20.11.2022].

BEHAR, RUTH 1997. *The Vulnerable Observer: Anthropology that Breaks your Heart*. Boston, MA: Beacon Press.

BERGMAN BLIX, STINA, & WETTERGREN, ÅSA 2015. The Emotional Labour of Gaining and Maintaining Access to the Field. *Qualitative research* 15, 6: 688–704.

BOHREN, MEGHAN; HOFMEYR, JUSTUS; SAKALA, CAROL; FUKU-ZAWA, RIEKO; & CUTHBERT, ANNA 2017. Continuous Support for Women during Childbirth. *The Cochrane Database of Systematic Reviews* 7, 7: CD003766.

BRADFIELD, ZOE, DUGGAN, RAVANI, HAUCK, YVONNE, & KELLY, MICHELLE 2018. Midwives Being 'With Woman': An Integrative Review. *Women and Birth* 31, 2: 143–152.

CANNELLA, GAILE S. & LINCOLN, YVONNA S. 2006. Predatory vs. Dialogic Ethics: Constructing an Illusion or Ethical Practice as the Core of Research methods. *Qualitative Inquiry* 13, 3: 315–335.

CARROLL, KATHERINE 2013. Infertile? The Emotional Labour of Sensitive and Feminist Research Methodologies. *Qualitative Research* 13, 5: 546–561.

CHADWICK, RACHELLE 2021. On the Politics of Discomfort. *Feminist Theory* 22, 4: 556–574.

DAVIS-FLOYD, ROBBIE 1994. The Technocratic Body: American Childbirth as Cultural Expression. *Social Science and Medicine*. 38, 8: 1125–1140.

DAVISS, BETTY-ANNE 2001. Reforming Birth and (Re)Making Midwifery in North America. In *Birth by Design*, eds. Raymond DeVries, Sirpa Wrede, Edwin R. Van Teijlingen, and Cecilia Benoit. New York: Routledge.

DICKSON, NONI 1996. A Theory of Caring for Midwifery. *Australian College of Midwives Incorporated Journal*, 9(2), 20–24.

DICKSON-SWIFT, VIRGINIA; JAMES, ERICA L.; KIPPEN, SANDRA & LIAMPUTTONG, PRANEE 2009. Researching Sensitive Topics: Qualitative Research as Emotion Work. *Qualitative research* 9, 1: 61–79.

DRIESSEN, ANNELIEKE; BORGSTROM, ERICA & COHN, SIMON 2021. Ways of 'Being With': Caring for Dying Patients at the Height of the COVID-19 Pandemic. *Anthropology in Action* 28, 1: 16–20.

ELLIS, CAROLYN 2007. Telling Secrets, Revealing Lives: Relational Ethics in Research with Intimate Others. *Qualitative inquiry* 13, 1: 3–29.

ELLINGSON, LAURA 1998. "Then You Know How I Feel": Empathy, Identification and Reflexivity in Fieldwork. *Qualitative Inquiry* 4, 4: 492–514.

FITZPATRICK, MOLLY 2020. Boundary Work in the Birthing Room: Doulas, Emotional Labour, and the Politics of Care. *Leiden Anthropology Blog*. https://www.leidenanthropologyblog.nl/articles/boundary-work-in-the-birthing-room-doulas-emotional-labour-and-the-politics-of-care [20.11.2022]

—— 2022. *Moral Becomings: The Affective Politics of Care in Midwifery Clinics in Bali, Indonesia*. PhD Thesis. Zurich: University of Zurich

FORD, ANDREA LILY 2020. Birthing From Within: Nature, Technology, and Self-Making in Silicon Valley Childbearing. *Cultural Anthropology* 35, 4: 602–63.

GARCIA, ANGELA 2010. *The Pastoral Clinic: Addiction and Dispossession along the Rio Grande*. Berkeley and Los Angeles: University of California Press.

GRUBER, KENNETH J.; CUPITO, SUSAN H. & DOBSON, CHRISTINA F. 2013. Impact of Doulas on Healthy Birth Outcomes. *The Journal of perinatal education* 22, 1: 49–58.

HALSE, CHRISTINE & HONEY, ANNE 2005. Unraveling Ethics: Illuminating the Moral Dilemmas of Research Ethics. *Signs: Journal of Women in Culture and Society* 30, 4: 2141–2162.

HOFMAN, EVA; GEURTS, SILVIA & SCHUL, KATARINA 2020. De Gynaecoloog Voelde zich Volledig Buitenspel Gezet. *NRC Handelsblad*, https://www.nrc.nl/nieuws/2020/09/22/de-gynaecoloog-voelde-zich-volledig-buitenspel-gezet-a4013125?t=1643902101 [03.02.2022].

HOLMES, MARY 2010. The Emotionalization of Reflexivity. *Sociology* 44, 1: 139–154.

KAUFMAN, KARYN 1993. Effective Control or Effective Care? *Birth* 20, 3: 156–157.

KNUDSEN, BRITTA & STAGE, CARSTEN 2015. 'Introduction: Affective Methodologies'. In KNUDSEN, BRITTA & STAGE, CARSTEN (eds) *Affective Methodologies: Developing Cultural Research Strategies for the Study of Affect*. London: Palgrave Macmillan: 1–24.

KOZHIMANNIL, KATY. B.; HARDEMAN, RACHEL R.; ALARID-ESCUDERO, FERNANDO; VOGELSANG, CARRIE. A.; BLAUER-PETERSON, CORI & HOWELL, ELIZABETH A. 2016. Modeling the Cost-effectiveness of Doula Care Associated with Reductions in Preterm Birth and Cesarean Delivery. *Birth* 43, 1: 20–27.

MACDONALD, MARGARET 2006. Gendered Expectations: Natural Bodies and Natural Births in the New Midwifery in Canada. *Medical Anthropology Quarterly* 20, 2: 235–256.

—— 2007. *At Work in the Field of Birth: Midwifery Narratives of Nature, Tradition, and Home*. Nashville, TN: Vanderbilt University Press.

MARXER, JILL 2022. Von Frau zu Frau Doulas und ihr "urweibliches Wissen". *Fakultativ*. https://www.theologie.uzh.ch/dam/jcr:d46afa97-b62b-42b4-bf7f-20ad34d56a4b/facultativ_2022_online.pdf [18.11.2022].

MENZFELD, MIRA 2022. Liminal Asymmetries: Making Sense of Transition Dynamics in Relations with Dying Persons, this issue

MEYERSON, COLLIER 2019. "A Landmark Bill Will Change the Way Doulas Do Business in New York." *Intelligencer*. https://nymag.com/intelligencer/2019/07/doula-certification-bill-in-new-york-state.html [07.10.2022].

MOL, ANNEMARIE; MOSER, INGUNN & POLS, JEANETTE 2010. Care: Putting Practice into Theory. In MOL, ANNEMARIE; MOSER, INGUNN & POLS, JEANETTE (eds) *Care in practice: On tinkering in clinics, homes and farms*. Bielefeld: Transcript: 7–19.

NEWLAND, LYNDA 2002. Of Paraji and Bidan: Hierarchies of Knowledge among Sundanese Midwives. In ROZARIO, SANTI & SAMUEL, GEOFFREY (eds) *The Daughters of Hariti: Childbirth and Female Healers of South and Southeast Asia*. London: Routledge: 256–279.

NIEHOF, ANKE 2014. Traditional Birth Attendants and the Problem of Maternal Mortality in Indonesia. *Pacific Affairs* 87, 4: 693–713.

NIEUWSUUR 2020. Waarom een Doula bij je Bevalling Wel/ Geen Goed Idee is, *Nieuwsuur* https://nos.nl/nieuwsuur/ artikel/2349980-waarom-een-doula-bij-je-bevalling-wel-geen-goed-idee-is [03.02.2022].

OAKLEY, ANN 1981. Interviewing Women: a Contradiction in Terms. In ROBERTS, HELEN (ed) *Doing Feminist Research*. London: Routledge and Kegan Paul: 30–61.

PASVEER, BERNIKE & AKRICH, MADELEINE 2001. Obstetrical Trajectories. On Training Women/Bodies for (Home)Birth. In DE VRIES, RAYMOND; WREDE, SIRPA; VAN TEIJLINGEN, EDWIN & BENOIT, CECILIA (eds) *Birth by Design. Pregnancy, Maternity Care and Midwifery in North America and Europe*. New York: Routledge: 229–242.

REHSMANN, JULIA 2019. Dancing Through the Perfect Storm: Encountering Illness and Death in the Field and Beyond. In STODULKA, THOMAS; DINKELAKER, SAMIA & THAJIB, FERDIANSYAH (eds) *Affective Dimensions of Fieldwork*. New York: Springer: 189 –200.

REHSMANN, JULIA & SIEGL, VERONIKA 2022. Ethnographic Explorations at the Beginnings and Ends of Life: An Introduction, *Curare* 45, 2: 5-14.

REINHARZ, SHULAMIT 1993. Neglected Voices and Excessive Demands in Feminist Research. *Qualitative Sociology* 16, 1: 69–76.

SAMPSON, HELEN; BLOOR, MICHAEL & FINCHAM, BEN 2008. A Price Worth Paying? Considering the 'Cost' of Reflexive Research Methods and the Influence of Feminist Ways of 'Doing'. *Sociology* 42, 5: 919–933.

SCHIAVENATO, STEPHANIE 2020. Birthing under Investigation. Covid-19, *Fieldsights*, May 1. https://culanth.org/fieldsights/birthing-under-investigation [28.02.22].

SKEIDE, ANNEKATRIN 2018. Witnessing as an Embodied Practice in German Midwifery Care. In KRAUSE, FRANZISKA & BOLDT, JOACHIM (eds) *Care in Healthcare: Reflections on Theory and Practice*. Cham: Springer: 191–209.

——— 2020. *Unnaturalizing Bodies: An Ethnographic Inquiry into Midwifery Care in Germany*. PhD Dissertation: University of Amsterdam.

STEVENSON, LISA 2014. *Life beside Itself: Imagining Care in the Canadian Arctic*. Oakland: University of California Press.

STOLLER, PAUL 2019. Afterword: A Return to the Story. In STODULKA, THOMAS; DINKELAKER, SAMIA & THAJIB, FERDIANSYAH (eds) *Affective Dimensions of Fieldwork*. New York: Springer: 347–352.

STRONG, ADRIENNE E. 2020. *Documenting Death: Maternal Mortality and the Ethics of Care in Tanzania*. Oakland, California: University of California Press.

THAJIB, FERDIANSYAH; DINKELAKER, SAMIA & STODULKA, THOMAS 2019. Introduction: Affective Dimensions of Fieldwork and Ethnography In STODULKA, THOMAS; DINKELAKER, SAMIA & THAJIB, FERDIANSYAH (eds) *Affective Dimensions of Fieldwork*. New York: Springer: 7–20.

VICKERS, ADRIAN 1989. *Bali: A Paradise Created*. Berkeley and Singapore: Periplus.

WETTERGREN, ÅSA 2015. How Do We Know What They Feel? In FLAM, HELENA & KLERES, JOCHEN (eds) *Methods of Exploring Emotions*. London and New York: Routledge: 115–124.

WIND, GITTE 2008. 'Negotiated Interactive Observation: Doing Fieldwork in Hospital Settings'. *Anthropology & Medicine* 15: 79–89.

YATES-DOERR, EMILY 2020. Antihero Care: On Fieldwork and Anthropology. *Anthropology and Humanism* 45, 2: 233–244.

Manuscript received: 11.03.2022
Manuscript accepted: 04.12.2022

MOLLY FITZPATRICK | PhD, is a postdoctoral researcher and lecturer at the department of social and cultural anthropology at the University of Zurich. She completed a bachelor degree in social anthropology and the research master social sciences at the University of Amsterdam. In 2021, she defended her PhD dissertation based on research in natural birthing clinics in Bali, Indonesia. In her dissertation, she explored how ideas about childbirth, motherhood, and care become imbued with moral significance for both midwives and birthing women, and how they negotiate those ideas in practice.

University of Zürich, ISEK – Social and Cultural Anthropology
Andreasstrasse 15, 8050 Zürich, Switzerland
molly.fitzpatrick@uzh.ch

Eine interdisziplinäre Betrachtung von „Ganzheitlichkeit" in Komplementär- und Alternativmedizin

JÜRGEN W. DOLLMANN

Abstract Komplementäre und alternative Medizinverfahren werden häufig mit dem Begriff der „Ganzheitlichkeit" unter Einbindung von „Körper, Geist und Seele" angeboten und rezipiert. Dieses Konzept, das im vorliegenden Beitrag im Zentrum steht, wird oft nicht nur als Abgrenzung zur Schulmedizin herangezogen, sondern häufig auch mit spirituellen Aspekten verbunden. Ein Grund dafür kann darin gesehen werden, dass viele komplementär- und alternativmedizinische Verfahren wie beispielsweise Ayurveda und Traditionelle Chinesische Medizin aus dem süd- bzw. ostasiatischen Bereich stammen und zum Teil aus religiösen bzw. philosophischen Traditionen abgeleitet werden. Der Autor, selbst Internist und Kulturwissenschaftler, führt historische und kulturwissenschaftliche Aspekte der „Ganzheitlichkeit" mit kognitions- und neurowissenschaftlichen Erkenntnissen zusammen. Eigene Feldforschungsergebnisse im Bereich des Ayurveda werden exemplarisch angeführt. Zur Integration dieser interdisziplinären Betrachtung dienen sogenannte Embodiment- oder Verkörperungstheorien, mit welchen die sinnliche Erfahrung von Akteurinnen und Akteuren im Untersuchungsfeld analysiert werden können. Der Ganzheitsbegriff kann aus dieser Perspektive als anschlussfähig an die spirituellen Aspekte der komplementär- und alternativmedizinischen Verfahren gesehen werden. Im Zentrum dieses Texts steht die Frage, wie und warum von Seiten der Patientinnen und Patienten eine „Ganzheit" erfahren und sinnlich erlebt werden kann. Die Frage nach der Wirksamkeit dieser Medizinverfahren wird nicht berührt. Die Positionalität des Verfassers ist explizit interdisziplinär und multiperspektivisch, wodurch angestrebt werden soll, blinde Flecken der verschiedenen Medizinverfahren aufzudecken. Die hier vorgenommene Methodentriangulation kann zu Ambiguitäten führen, die jedoch als Diskussionsanregung zwischen kultur- und naturwissenschaftlichen Perspektiven verstanden werden sollen. In einem Resümee werden Anregungen gegeben, die helfen könnten, dem wechselseitigen Ausgrenzungsdiskurs der unterschiedlichen Heilsysteme entgegenzuwirken. Das Ziel ist die weitere Förderung einer Integrativen Medizin.

Schlagwörter Komplementär- und Alternativmedizin – Evidenzbasierte Medizin – Ganzheitsmedizin – Integrative Medizin – Embodiment – Spiritualität.

Einleitung: Die Entdifferenzierung von Medizin und Religion

Seit mehreren Jahrzehnten ist auf dem Feld der Medizin nicht nur in Deutschland, sondern allgemein in der „westlichen" Welt, empirisch eine Zunahme von komplementär- und alternativmedizinischen Heilmethoden (Complementary and Alternative Medicine, im Folgenden mit CAM abgekürzt), zu registrieren (FRASS, STRASSL, FRIEHS, MÜLLNER, KUNDI & KAYE 2012: 45–56; DILGER & SCHNEPF 2020: 13–14). Unter CAM werden Medizinverfahren subsumiert, welche nicht der landeseigenen traditionellen oder konventionellen medizinischen Lehre entsprechen (WHO 2019: 28). Die zunehmende Koexistenz der CAM mit der akademischen Medizin wird oft unter dem Begriff Neuer Medizinischer Pluralismus gefasst (JÜTTE 2017: 7). Der Medizinhistoriker ROBERT JÜTTE betont, dass auch in dieser Koexistenz aktuell die wechselseitigen Ausgrenzungsdiskurse noch anhalten, obwohl sich die CAM „wachsender Beliebtheit in der Bevölkerung erfreuen" (2017: 6). Diese immer noch anhaltenden Diskurse haben vielfältige Perspektiven, wobei auch die hegemoniale Macht der akademischen Medizin eine wesentliche Rolle spielt (PATTATHU 2015: 332). Von Seiten der CAM wird in diesem Ausgrenzungsdiskurs der Begriff Schulmedizin oft pejorativ verwendet, der Mensch werde in dieser akademisch geprägten Medizin nur fragmentiert wahrgenommen (BÖKER 2003: A 24–A 26–27; DOLLMANN 2021: 83). Als Selbstbezeichnung der akademischen Medizin hat sich der Begriff Evidenzbasierte Medizin etabliert. Dadurch soll betont werden, dass sich dieses Therapieverfahren an den anerkanntesten derzeit verfügbaren externen klinischen Evidenzstudien orientieren muss (SACKETT, ROSENBERG, GRAY, HAYNES & RICHARDSON 1996: 71). Die vorliegende Arbeit greift – jenseits der institutionellen und gesundheitspolitischen Dimensionen – eine spezielle Semantik auf, welche in diesen Diskursen eine zentrale Rolle spielt: Das in der Selbstverortung der CAM häufig anzutreffende Narrativ bezieht sich auf eine „Ganzheitlichkeit" unter Berücksichtigung von „Körper, Geist und Seele", wobei oft auch spirituelle Aspekte angeführt werden. Dies wird weiter unten in dieser Arbeit exemplarisch aus Internetrecherchen und Feldforschungsergebnissen ersichtlich.

Im Feld der Religionen kommt es seit vielen Jahren zu einer Zunahme von Gruppierungen, die religiöse Rituale zur kurativen Behandlung von Krankheiten vornehmen (LÜDDECKENS 2012: 290). Beispiele finden sich in pfingstlich-charismatischen Gemeinden u. a. in Nordamerika und Europa. Diese beiden zunächst unabhängig erscheinenden Phänomene – der Seelenaspekt und spirituelle Semantiken in vielen CAM-Verfahren einerseits und die Heilungsrituale innerhalb bestimmter religiöser Gruppierungen andererseits – werden religionswissenschaftlich als „Entdifferenzierung von Medizin und Religion" seit Jahren analysiert (LÜDDECKENS 2012: 288–297). Historisch orientierte sich der Begriff Heilung spätestens ab dem 18. Jahrhundert an wissenschaftlichen Erkenntnissen in einer akademischen medizinischen Ausbildung, während der Begriff Heil im Bereich von Religionen verortet wurde. Diese Ausdifferenzierung der beiden gesellschaftlichen Subsysteme Medizin und Religion ging mit einer sogenannten Medikalisierung einher (LÜDDECKENS 2012: 284): Ehemals im religiösen oder sozialen Umfeld gesuchte Abweichungen von einer angenommenen Normalität wie zum Beispiel Kinderlosigkeit oder Epilepsie wurden zum Gegenstand wissenschaftlich zu untersuchender Krankheiten. Den Ursachen, inwiefern seit ca. 50 Jahren diese Grenze zwischen Religion und Medizin innerhalb oben genannter

Diskurse wieder fließender geworden ist, soll im Folgenden nachgegangen werden. Durch Klärung der Hintergründe dieser Entdifferenzierung kann meines Erachtens der Ausgrenzungsdiskurs zwischen CAM und Schulmedizin einem besseren gegenseitigen Verständnis weichen. Die im Titel stehende „Ganzheitlichkeit" von CAM-Verfahren soll im Folgenden unter historischen, anthropologischen[1] und medizinischen Aspekten beleuchtet werden, da „Ganzheitlichkeit" – wie zu zeigen sein wird – ein Schlüsselbegriff in der Gemengelage zwischen CAM und Evidenzbasierter Medizin darstellt. Der Ganzheitsanspruch wird im Folgenden näher erörtert und dessen Zusammenhang zu einem rezenten Spiritualitätsbegriff analysiert.

Historische und religiös-weltanschauliche Hintergründe

Der Anspruch einer Betrachtung des kranken Menschen als ein „Ganzes" ist keine Forderung, die erst im 20. Jahrhundert aufkam. Schon ERASMUS VON ROTTERDAM (~1469–1536), ein niederländischer Gelehrter des Renaissance-Humanismus, forderte, dass der Arzt nicht nur für den Körper Sorge tragen solle, welcher der „wertlosere Teil des Menschen" sei. Er solle dagegen „den ganzen Menschen" (ERASMUS 2008: 39) im Blick haben. SAMUEL HAHNEMANN (1755–1843), Begründer der Homöopathie, bezeichnet in seinem *Organon der Heilkunst* den kranken Menschen als „ein Ganzes" (HAHNEMANN 2001: 67).

Außerhalb religiöser Traditionen nicht nur den Menschen, sondern das gesamte Universum unter einem holistischen, „ganzheitlichen" Aspekt neu zu betrachten, kam jedoch in der westlichen Welt erst im 19. Jahrhundert auf: In dieser Hochphase der Kolonialisierung erforschten westliche Orientalisten asiatische Religionen/Philosophien[2] wie beispielsweise die buddhistischen und hinduistischen Traditionen. Intellektuelle antiklerikale Kreise im Westen, geprägt von der Aufklärung, suchten in dieser Zeit Alternativen zum Christentum, welches als dogmatisch angesehen wurde (KING 1999: 122). Der hinduistische Mönch SWAMI VIVEKANANDA (1863–1902) referierte im ersten Weltparlament der Religionen 1893 in Chicago über die religiöse/philosophische Tradition namens advaita vedanta, die er als Hinduismus dem Christentum als gleichberechtigt entgegenstellte (BERGUNDER 2012: 99). Hinter dieser von VIVEKANANDA vertretenen Tradition steht die Grundannahme der Identität eines Selbst mit dem Absoluten (FIGL 2003: 317) und somit nicht ein dualistisches, sondern ein monistisches Weltbild. Damit ist plausibel, dass diese Darstellung in antireligiösen intellektuellen Kreisen anerkannt wurde, da sie dem christlichen Dualismus von Gott und Mensch entgegenstand. Aber auch von liberalen Christen wurde VIVEKANANDAS advaita vedanta anerkannt: Der Philosoph Max Müller sah darin eine Möglichkeit, eine Verbindung zum Christentum, einen Christlichen Vedanta herzustellen (HANEGRAAFF, 2007: 122). Ein weiterer attraktiver Aspekt aus Sicht der Orientalisten war VIVEKANANDAS Aussage, dass alles Wissen auf Erfahrung beruhe (BERGUNDER 2016: 110–111). In der Folge wurde somit von manchen Protagonisten ein neues Verhältnis von Religion und Wissenschaft konstruiert: Die beiden Entitäten würden lediglich zwei Dimensionen menschlicher Existenz entsprechen: einer spirituellen und einer rationalen. Der Begriff Spiritualität ist zwar europäischer Herkunft: Das Adjektiv spiritualis stand im Mittelalter u. a. im Mönchtum für eine geistliche Bindung, im Gegensatz zu einer Bindung an die materielle, aus der Sicht des Christentums auch zeitlich begrenzte, Welt (BOCHINGER 1995: 378). VIVEKANANDA integrierte diesen Begriff jedoch in seine Darstellung des advaita vedanta, den er im „Hinduismus"[3] verortet:

> Touch him on spirituality, on religion, on God, on the soul, on the Infinite, on spiritual freedom, and I assure you, the lowest peasant in India is better informed on these subjects than many a so-called philosopher in other lands (VIVEKANANDA 1958a: 148).
>
> With the Hindus you will find one national idea – spirituality. In no other religion, in no other sacred books of the world, will you find so much energy spent in defining the idea of God (VIVEKANANDA 1958b: 372).

Die Rezeption von VIVEKANANDAS advaita vedanta wurde später teils als neo-Hinduismus, neo-Vedanta oder neo-Advaita bezeichnet (KING 1999: 135).

Die Vorstellung des ceylonesischen Theravada Buddhismus, geprägt von ANAGARIKA DHARMA

PALA (1864–1933) auf dem Weltparlament der Religionen, stellt eine weitere Perspektive dar, welche im Verlauf des 20. Jahrhunderts Bedeutung erlangte: Auch DHARMAPALA sah keine Trennung von Buddhismus und Wissenschaft, für ihn war der Buddhismus eine wissenschaftliche Religion (BERGUNDER 2016: 114). Von der Theosophischen Gesellschaft wurde Ende des 19. und Anfang des 20. Jahrhunderts schließlich eine nicht-institutionalisierte holistische Spiritualität dem abgelehnten oder kritisch gesehenen Christentum entgegengesetzt. Von hier aus gibt es eine Rezeptionslinie bis zur New-Age-Bewegung in den 1960er Jahren, wo es zur Popularisierung dieser spirituellen, „ganzheitlichen" Weltanschauungen kam (BOCHINGER 1995: 137) Die New-Age-Bewegung war sicher nicht homogen, aber deren holistische Weltsicht beeinflusste zahlreiche gesellschaftliche Diskurse des 20. Jahrhunderts und wirkt auch im 21. Jahrhundert: Friedensbewegung, ökologisches Denken und eine „ganzheitliche" Medizin wurden zu populären Themen in den Medien und prägten mehrere Generationen. Der Kulturhistoriker WOUTER HANEGRAAFF bemerkt hierzu:

> The consequences for our general culture will be no less momentous than those which resulted from the scientific revolution. Thus, the idea of the emerging „new paradigm" is the scientific parallel of the New Age idea (2007: 35).

Erst in der zweiten Hälfte des 20. Jahrhunderts kam es infolge dieser Popularisierung zur breiteren Wahrnehmung beispielsweise der Traditionellen Chinesischen Medizin (TCM) und der Akupunktur. Hinter diesem Medizinverfahren steht die Weltanschauung des Daoismus mit den ineinander verschränkten Kräften Yin und Yang, die nicht nur im Körper, sondern im gesamten Universum wirksam seien (JÜTTE 1996: 263). Ebenso wurde aus der hinduistischen Tradition im Westen der Ayurveda populär, der auch von einem fluiden, mit der natürlichen und sozialen Umwelt verflochtenen lebendigen Körper ausgeht (LANGFORD 2002: 11). Historisch besteht somit eine enge Verbindung von „ganzheitlicher" Heilung und Spiritualität.[4] Der zunächst aus dem Christentum stammende Begriff Spiritualität wandelte sich somit im Laufe des 20. Jahrhunderts und wird heute überwiegend als alternative, nicht institutionalisierte und individualisierte Religiosität verstanden (KING 2007: 320). Gegenläufig zu den Kirchenaustritten der letzten Jahrzehnte wird empirisch eine Zunahme von alternativen Religionen bzw. Spiritualitäten festgestellt, wobei auffällig ist, dass in diesen neuen Bewegungen der Körper, rituelle Handlungen und das individuelle Erleben eine große Rolle spielen (HEELAS & WOODHEAD 2005: 3–9). PAUL HEELAS und LINDA WOODHEAD (2005: 8) fanden in ihren empirischen Untersuchungen, dass sich im Feld der CAM überwiegend Akteure und Akteurinnen finden, die sich als spirituell bezeichnen. Sie prägten hierfür den Begriff des Holistischen Milieus, den sie synonym mit New-Age-Spiritualität verwenden. Der Begriff des Holistischen Milieus wurde breit rezipiert und steht auch bei anderen Autoren für die „alternative therapeutische und spirituelle Szene" (HÖLLINGER & TRIPOLD 2012: 11). Die Entdifferenzierung von Religion und Medizin der vergangenen Jahrzehnte in der westlichen Welt kann unter diesen Aspekten eine weitere Erklärung finden: Wenn eine disparate, unübersichtliche Gesellschaft allgemeine Sinnstiftung weder über philosophische Ideen noch über religiöse Orientierung im traditionellen Sinne mehr liefert, kann der Körper zum „Medium von Ganzheitserfahrungen oder besser Ganzheitskonstruktionen" werden (MOHN 2007: 68). In der Religionssoziologie wird thematisiert, dass der eigene Körper „sakralisiert" werde (HERO 2009: 206; HOUTMAN & AUPERS 2008), Gesundheit werde so zum höchsten Gut, Ärzte und Ärztinnen, Heiler und Heilerinnen lösen traditionelle Seelsorger und Seelsorgerinnen ab. Das individuelle Erleben, die Erfahrung von „Ganzheit" und die spirituellen Aspekte im Ayurveda lassen sich auch vor diesem Hintergrund interpretieren, darauf wird weiter unten eingegangen. Bevor das Problem der Ganzheitlichkeit näher analysiert wird, muss ein Problem des Begriffes Spiritualität geklärt werden: Es kann aktuell keine allgemeingültige Definition für Spiritualität formuliert werden. Der Begriff wird je nach soziokulturellem Kontext divers und teilweise widersprüchlich interpretiert, wie es auch aus einer interdisziplinär konzipierten Studie hervorgeht:

> Our results clearly show that there is no single notion of „spirituality," but a broad semantic diversity. This is mirrored in particular by our first result, the system of no less than 44 categories which were necessary to capture the various topoi, symbolizations, and meanings of our respondents' definitions. It is probably this multitude of understandings that causes the often stated „fuzziness" of the term „spirituality." (EISENMANN, KLEIN, SWHAJOR-BIESEMANN, DREXELIUS, KELLER & STREIB 2016: 145).

Die Autorinnen und Autoren konnten durch eine Hauptkomponentenanalyse ihrer Statistik aus den 44 Kategorien 10 relevante Dimensionen herausarbeiten (EISENMANN, KLEIN, SWHAJOR-BIESEMANN, DREXELIUS, KELLER & STREIB 2016: 136–138). Die gefundenen Kategorien resultieren aus einem Vergleich von Erhebungen in Deutschland und den USA. Da in der vorliegenden Arbeit die charakteristischen, rezenten Zuschreibungen zu Spiritualität im Holistischen Milieu deutscher Ayurveda-Einrichtungen stehen, bezieht sich der folgende Cluster auf die Literaturergebnisse zu diesem Milieu, die Erhebungen der eigenen Feldstudien inklusive der angeführten Internetrecherchen zu den Ayurvedaeinrichtungen und die oben angeführten historischen Hintergründe (DOLLMANN 2021: 69–72, 110–161). Charakteristisch für Spiritualität in dem genannten Feld ist eine Betonung der subjektiven Erfahrung, die „ganzheitliche" Betrachtung aller Phänomene, die Fluidität und häufige Bricolage aus verschiedensten Traditionen, jedoch meist die Ablehnung von Dogmatik und christlich-religiösen Traditionen. Das letztere Argument trifft überwiegend auf Europa zu, in den USA findet man aus historischen Gründen häufiger die christlich verortete Selbsteinschätzung als spirituell (AMMERMAN 2013: 266–268). Selbstverständlich gibt es zu den Semantiken dieser Auswahl an Zuschreibungen auch gegensätzliche Positionen, aber die Tendenz der Zunahme einer subjektivistischen, nicht-christlichen, holistischen Spiritualität geht auch aus den Argumenten der bisher schon angeführten Autorinnen und Autoren hervor.

Ein Problem hinter der angenommen „Ganzheitlichkeit"

Die Begriffe Spiritualität und „Ganzheitlichkeit" sind eng verschränkt, dabei zeigt sich eine große Variation sowohl des Verständnisses als auch der Verwendung des Begriffes der „Ganzheitlichkeit" in unterschiedlichen soziokulturellen Kontexten. Der Begriff wird in dem hier behandelten Feld des Ayurveda nahezu regelmäßig betont (Dollmann: 117–118). Jedoch auch im weiteren Feld der holistischen Gesundheitsbewegungen werde „ganzheitliches" Denken zum Paradigma erhoben (JESERICH 2010: 206). Die Ärztin und Wissenschaftsjournalistin RENATE JÄCKLE begründet die Häufigkeit und Popularität des Begriffes im Bereich von Heilung auch mit einer hohen Zahl an populären Ratgebern und einer „Fülle von Veranstaltungen" (JÄCKLE 1985: 80). Die Autorin interpretiert die Zunahme des Ganzheitsbegriffes im CAM-Bereich als Reaktion auf die Krise in der Schulmedizin, wo dem Patienten oder der Patientin nicht mehr ausreichend Zeit entgegengebracht werde (JÄCKLE 1985: 60–70). Der Begriff der „Ganzheit" werde zunehmend „inflationär verwendet" (JÄCKLE 1985: 62). Dass sich in der Schulmedizin ein Reduktionismus ausgebreitet habe, indem der Patient oder die Patientin nur noch fragmentiert wahrgenommen werde, wurde oben schon expliziert. Insofern darf „Ganzheitsmedizin" im hier vorliegenden soziokulturellen Kontext der rezenten CAM-Verfahren in Deutschland als Gegenentwurf zur zugeschrieben fraktionierenden Schulmedizin aufgefasst werden. „Ganzheitlichkeit" kann in dem hier untersuchten Feld für die Erfassung des „ganzen" Menschen stehen, ohne Vernachlässigung von Teilen, die mit dem Menschen untrennbar in Verbindung stehen und evtl. für die Ätiologie von Krankheiten (mit)verantwortlich sind. Diese Formulierung orientiert sich am Holismusanspruch, wie er in der Rezeption der New-Age-Bewegung auch für die Medizin gefordert wird. Der Quantenphysiker FRITJOF CAPRA, der auch als „New-Age-Autor" (BERGUNDER 2020: 116) bezeichnet wird, schreibt im Vorwort zu einem Buch über „ganzheitliche" Medizin, am wichtigsten seien in diesem Zusammenhang: „[...] Selbsterfahrung, spirituelles Bewußtsein und eine ganzheitliche Sicht von Gesundheit und Heilung"[5] (CAPRA 1985: 12). Zu diesem spirituellen Bewusstsein des Menschen bemerkt er, dass „[...] der Begriff des transzendenten menschlichen Geistes verstanden wird als Bewußtseinsform, in der sich der Mensch mit dem Kosmos als ganzem (sic!) verbunden fühlt" (CAPRA 1985: 9).

Dies äußert CAPRA explizit im Zusammenhang mit „ganzheitlicher" Medizin, und auch hier wird „Ganzheitlichkeit" mit Spiritualität verbunden. Diese „Ganzheitlichkeit" lässt sich jedoch mit naturwissenschaftlichen Methoden nicht operationalisieren: In CAM-Verfahren wie Ayurveda wird die postulierte „Ganzheitlichkeit" häufig mit der Berücksichtigung von „Körper, Geist und Seele" in Zusammenhang gebracht (weiter unten folgen Beispiele). Der Begriff einer „Seele", welche zusätzlich zum „Geist" behandelt werden solle, ist nach meiner Auffassung dem religiösen oder spirituellen Bereich zuordenbar und lässt sich empirisch nicht fassen. Ein Problem der „Ganzheitlichkeit" in der Medizin kann auch darin gesehen werden, dass weder CAM-Verfahren noch die Evidenzbasierte Medizin den „ganzen Menschen" im Sinne der obigen Formulierung erfassen können. Jedes Medizinsystem hat seine eigenen spezifischen Grundprinzipien: In der TCM ist dies beispielsweise eine angenommene Energie QI, welche in den Meridianen unter den Kräften Yin und Yang fließt. Krankheiten entstehen in dieser Ontologie aus dem Ungleichgewicht dieser Kräfte, die entsprechenden Erkenntnismaßnahmen zur Diagnosestellung müssen sich somit am Erkennen dieses Ungleichgewichtes orientieren (JÜTTE 1996: 263–264). Im Ayurveda gehören dagegen die drei sogenannten Doshas (Vata, Pitta und Kapha) zum spezifischen Grundprinzip: Diese Doshas – man kann sie als eine Art Konstitutionstypen verstehen – regulieren im ayurvedischen Denken die psychischen und somatischen Lebensprozesse, sind bei jedem Menschen vorhanden und werden schon von Geburt an in einer bestimmten individuellen Mischkonstellation mitgebracht (CHOPRA 2012: 11). Dosha bedeutet wörtlich übersetzt „Verderber" (CHOPRA 2012: 11), was sich wie folgt erklärt: Eine Störung ihrer Homöostase führt zu Krankheiten mit entsprechenden Affektionen auch der strukturellen Anteile des Organismus. Diagnoseverfahren müssen sich somit an den Charakteristika und Homöostase-Störungen der Doshas orientieren. Es ist ersichtlich, dass je nach Ontologie ein eingeschränkter Fokus auf Spezifika des kranken Menschen vorliegt: Wissen kann es auch in den CAM-Verfahren immer nur als Wissen um etwas Bestimmtes geben, nie als Wissen von einem „Ganzen" (ZINSER 2005: 36). Der eingeschränkte Fokus betrifft selbstverständlich auch die Evidenzbasierte Medizin: Die ontologischen Ausgangspunkte der Diagnostik sind beispielsweise die Organe oder der Stoffwechsel. In den Fachbereichen der Psychosomatischen Medizin oder der Psychiatrie stehen die Psyche und damit auch der soziale Kontext im Fokus der Diagnostik. Eine „ganzheitliche" Betrachtung ist auch aus praktischen Gründen nicht erreichbar: „Ganzheitliche" Diagnostik gemäß obiger Formulierung würde voraussetzen, dass anamnestisch die gesamte psychosoziale Entwicklung kranker Personen von Geburt an eruiert werden müsste, ebenso wie alle anderen umweltkontextualen Faktoren. Weiterhin müssten alle machbaren Laborwerte erhoben werden und alle Organe einschließlich des vollständigen Zahnstatus und des Zentralnervensystems untersucht werden. Alle der möglichen bildgebenden Verfahren wie Sonographie, Radiologie inklusive Computertomographie und Kernspintomographie oder Koronarangiographie müssten durchgeführt werden. Bei dieser Aufzählung sind noch viele weitere Untersuchungstechniken unterschlagen worden. Diese Fülle an Diagnostik würde evtl. eine Annäherung an eine zu erstrebende „ganzheitliche" Sicht auf den Patienten bzw. die Patientin aus naturwissenschaftlich-empirischer Perspektive darstellen. Es ist aber evident, dass ein solches Vorgehen unmöglich, das heißt den jeweiligen Problemkomplexen des kranken Menschen unangemessen und weiterhin weder zeitlich noch finanziell praktikabel wäre. Diese „Ganzheitlichkeit" ist somit nicht einlösbar, auch wenn schulmedizinische Hausärzte und Hausärztinnen ihre Patienten und Patientinnen einschließlich deren Familie oft seit Jahrzehnten kennen und oft über zahlreiche Hausbesuche auch häusliche Problemsituationen in Augenschein nehmen konnten. ZINSER (2005: 36) betont in einer Frobenius-Vorlesung polemisch, dass diejenigen, die von „Ganzheit" reden, nicht wüssten, von was sie reden: Wissen setze immer Differenzierung und Abgrenzung voraus. Auf diese Polemik kann man jedoch verzichten, wenn die kulturwissenschaftlichen und naturwissenschaftlichen Perspektiven nicht gegeneinander ausgespielt werden, sondern in einen Diskurs treten. Der folgende Abschnitt soll einen Beitrag zu diesem Diskurs leisten.

Die Wahrnehmung einer „Ganzheitlichkeit" über verkörpertes Erleben

Unabhängig von der dargelegten Problematik einer „Ganzheitsmedizin" werden viele CAM-Verfahren unter diesem Konzept angeboten und rezipiert (DOLLMANN 2021: 86–88). Würden sich Patienten und Patientinnen in einer überwiegenden Zahl innerhalb dieser Therapieverfahren jedoch nicht „ganzheitlich" behandelt fühlen, wären die Verfahren unter dem Konzept „Ganzheitlichkeit" aus dem Markt der Heilangebote verschwunden. Sie nehmen jedoch zu, wie oben schon belegt. Wie ist das Erleben einer „Ganzheitlichkeit" zu erklären? Bevor auf diese Frage eingegangen wird, muss Folgendes noch einmal klar ausgedrückt werden: Es geht in diesem Artikel nicht um die medizinische Wirksamkeit von CAM-Verfahren, hierzu liegen zahlreiche unterschiedlich konzipierte Studien vor. Hier geht es ausschließlich um die Frage, warum und wodurch sich Akteure und Akteurinnen als „ganzheitlich" behandelt fühlen.

Sogenannte Embodiment-Theorien zeigen, dass wir unsere Umwelt primär sinnlich perzipieren, und zwar vor jeder analytischen Trennung von Subjekt und Objekt, von Körper und Geist (CSORDAS 1990: 6–39). Es sind also nicht objektiv gegebene Phänomene der Außenwelt, die „wahr"genommen werden: Allein schon physikalisch können wir nur einen Ausschnitt elektromagnetischer Wellenlängen als sichtbares Licht wahrnehmen, genauso besteht eine Begrenzung in der Perzeption von Schallfrequenzen (KAISER 2018: 2.2.1). Weiterhin nehmen wir die Umwelt zu einem gegebenen Zeitpunkt immer nur aus einer Perspektive wahr, und dies nicht nur vor einem optischen Horizont, sondern auch vor einem je individuellen Wissens- und Erfahrungshorizont. Um handlungsfähig zu sein kommt es – aus dieser Perspektive – über eine konstruktive Leistung unseres mentalen Systems zu einer „perzeptiven Synthese" unserer Sinneseindrücke und damit erst zur Wahrnehmung einer Kohärenz, einer „Ganzheit" (MERLEAU-PONTY 1964: 16; MOHR 2005: 621). Die sinnliche Perzeption und deren perzeptive Synthese sind jedoch nicht essentialistisch gegeben oder etwa eindeutig naturalistisch determiniert, sondern auch kulturell geprägt. Beispiele für diese Mechanismen sind z. B.

optische Täuschungen wie das sogenannte Kanizsa-Dreieck: Die früheren sinnlichen Erfahrungen geometrischer Figuren lassen uns in dieser optischen Darstellung ein weißes Dreieck wahrnehmen, obwohl „objektiv" nur drei schwarze Kreisausschnitte vorliegen (KAISER 2018: 2.2.1.3 Abb. 4). Diese Prozesse laufen weitgehend unbewusst ab, die sinnlichen Eindrücke werden von uns deswegen meist als vollständige und wirklichkeitsgetreue Abbilder der Außenwelt erlebt, obwohl sie teilweise illusionär sein könnten. Ein weiterer Faktor zum Verständnis unserer Perzeption sind die sogenannten „sensomotorischen Kontingenzen" (O'REGAN & NOÉ 2013: 332–342): Die visuelle „Wahr"nehmung beispielsweise ist nicht allein über die Sehrinde im Okzipitallappen zu erklären: Wir sehen ein Objekt zunächst nur aus einer Perspektive. Das „Rund-Sein" eines Glases wird situativ gleichzeitig durch den Tastsinn bestätigt, „begriffen". Ein gutes Beispiel für die Bedeutung dieser visuellen sensomotorischen Kontingenz belegen Aufzeichnungen von Menschen, die mit einer angeborenen Linsentrübung blind auf die Welt kamen und die durch eine Operation erstmals sehen können: Nach dem Eingriff sind sie überrascht, dass eine runde Münze, wenn sie in der Hand gedreht wird, scheinbar ihre Form ändert und über die Projektion der Netzhaut elliptisch erscheint (O'REGAN & NOÉ 2013: 336). Das „Rund-Sein" wird erst in der multimodalen, sensomotorischen Wahrnehmung realisiert und in der Zusammenarbeit mit der Haptik erschlossen. Dieses Phänomen betrifft je nach Kontext auch andere Sinnesmodalitäten. Menschen erfassen die Umwelt somit nicht nur sensorisch multimodal, sondern gleichzeitig untrennbar in ihrer motorischen Aktivität über verschaltete Netzwerke, die auch die Mechano- und Propriozeptoren der Körperperipherie integrieren. Die Perzeption multimodaler sensorischer Eindrücke löst erst ein „ganzheitliches" Erleben aus (KOCH 2007: 161). Der Blick über ein Fernglas auf den Meeresstrand unterscheidet sich radikal von dem Erleben, an diesem Strand zu stehen: Der optische Eindruck von Meer, Himmel und Sonne wird über die Fußsohlen mit dem haptischen Erspüren der Struktur und der Temperatur des Sandes und über die Haut mit der Windprise verbunden, olfaktorisch wird der Salzgeruch wahrgenommen. Diese vielfältigen

Eindrücke, in unserem Nervensystem multimodal vernetzt abgespeichert, erklären auch, dass ein bestimmter Geruch plötzlich eine längst verschüttete Kindheitserinnerung auslösen kann. Die hier kurz zusammengefassten Erkenntnisse führen zu einem tieferen Verständnis der Erfahrung einer erstrebten „Ganzheitlichkeit" und lassen sich, wie weiter unten zu zeigen ist, auf den Bereich Ayurveda übertragen. Die Frage, warum und wie sowohl „Ganzheitlichkeit" als auch Spiritualität erfahren werden können, steht ja im Zentrum dieses Artikels. Der Erfahrungsbegriff muss zuvor noch näher thematisiert werden: Eine Erfahrung „an sich" ist nicht operationalisierbar, sie ist ein subjektiv empfundenes Phänomen, das über das Bewusstsein erst zur Versprachlichung kommen kann (KNOBLAUCH 2003: 32–47). Damit kommen Körper und Wissen zusammen, wofür der Begriff des „Körperwissens" (KOCH 2007: 279) steht. ANNE KOCH kommt „[...] zu dem Ergebnis, dass Körperwissen ein nonpropositionales Wissen ist, insofern es inkommensurabel und nicht analog zu propositionalen Arten des Wissens, z. B. sprachlichem Wissen, ist" (2007: 279).

Die Erfahrung – z. B. von „Ganzheitlichkeit" oder Spiritualität – als ein subjektiv empfundenes Phänomen, kann nach der Versprachlichung in qualitativen Interviews erfasst werden. Die Versprachlichung ist somit als eine Konstruktion erster Ordnung von Seiten der Akteure und Akteurinnen aufzufassen (KNOBLAUCH 2003: 32–33). Die Einbettung in eine wissenschaftliche Theorie von Seiten des Forschers oder der Forscherin entspricht dann einer Konstruktion zweiter Ordnung. Wegen dieser Konstruktionen und den damit evtl. verbundenen Problemen der Validität wird in dieser Arbeit eine interdisziplinäre Triangulation vorgenommen: Die Triangulation entspricht der wissenschaftlichen Betrachtung eines Gegenstandsbereiches von mindestens zwei Seiten (KNOBLAUCH 2003: 165–166). In dieser Arbeit ist der Gegenstandsbereich die „Ganzheitlichkeit" und die damit oft verbundene Spiritualität. Die Triangulation betreffend stehen auf der einen Seite die kulturwissenschaftlichen Methoden z. B. der Feldforschung und der Historiographie, auf der anderen Seite die kognitions- und neurowissenschaftlichen Erkenntnisse sowie die Embodiment-Theorien. Durch die Triangulation kann gemäß Knoblauch die Validität und Reliabilität empirischer Untersuchungen bekräftigt werden, wenn sich Synergien ergeben (KNOBLAUCH 2003: 163–166).

„Ganzheitlichkeit" und „Spiritualität": Ayurveda als Paradigma für CAM

Der Ayurveda war schon historisch auf dem indischen Subkontinent ständigen Transformationen unterworfen, was inneren Entwicklungen, ökologischen Veränderungen und der immerwährenden Veränderung von Religion und Kultur zuzuschreiben ist (SMITH & WUJASTYK 2008: 6). Ayurveda hat sich im Rahmen der britischen Kolonialisierung jedoch gegenläufig zur späteren Rezeption in der westlichen Welt transformiert,[6] hier können nur einzelne, charakteristische Befunde herausgegriffen werden: In Indien kam es nach der Kolonialisierung zunächst aus anti-britischen Motiven zu einer Betonung von spirituellen Aspekten des Ayurveda, die später jedoch einer „Resäkularisierung" wich (KOCH 2005: 27). Diese Entwicklung ist vor dem Hintergrund der von den Briten eingeführten neuen Methoden und Technologien für Diagnose und Forschung zu verstehen und kann als „biomedicalization" (SMITH & WUJASTYK 2008: 8) von Ayurveda bezeichnet werden. Dementgegen habe die Wahrnehmung von Ayurveda als Teil der vedischen Literatur und die damit verbundene Einbettung in die hinduistische Tradition im Rahmen der westlichen Ausbreitung sich „[...] zu einer Strömung, die neue „ganzheitliche" Deutungsmuster und Lebensweisen entwickelt [...]" ausgeweitet (KOCH 2005: 27). Die Autorin bezeichnet diese Transformationen als „Spiritualisierung eines Heilwissens" (KOCH 2005: 21). Dieselbe Autorin argumentiert in einer anderen Veröffentlichung: „Was den Ayurveda im Westen so attraktiv macht, ist seine Aufmachung: er wird nicht lediglich als Medizin, sondern als spirituelles Sinnangebot offeriert" (KOCH 2006: 170). Dazu gibt es empirische Befunde: In einer Untersuchung in Deutschland wurden 140 Patienten und Patientinnen sowie Therapierende befragt: 72,9 % der Befragten verbanden Ayurveda mit Spiritualität, es war zudem eine Affinität der Befragten zu Hinduismus und Buddhismus nachweisbar (KESSLER, WISCHNEWSKY, MICHALSEN, EISENMANN & MELZER 2013: 5–7). Dass in derselben Er-

hebung 94,6 % der Teilnehmenden Ayurveda als Medizinsystem sahen, ist kein Widerspruch: Aus der oben explizierten Geschichte der Spiritualität ließ sich ableiten, dass im Holistischen Milieu Spiritualität und Wissenschaft als kompatibel gesehen werden. In der genannten Studie sahen 76 % der Teilnehmenden den medizinischen Aspekt von Ayurveda als wichtiger im Verhältnis zu religiösen oder spirituellen Aspekten. Es gibt ebenso Verfechter und Verfechterinnen eines reinen wissenschaftlichen Status von Ayurveda, nach denen religiöse und spirituelle Spekulationen als nicht systemimmanent betrachtet werden. Als Beispiel in Deutschland wird ANANDA SAMIR CHOPRA gesehen, der seine Arbeit in der von ihm geleiteten Ayurveda-Abteilung in Kassel wissenschaftlich als medizinische Disziplin vertritt (PATTATHU 2015: 315–316, 324). Auch für ANTONY PATTATHU stellt Ayurveda ein „ganzheitliches" System dar. Der Autor betont, dass die jeweilige Zuordnung im „Spannungsfeld Religion und Medizin" (PATTATHU 2015: 301) in Deutschland von ökonomischen und rechtlichen Strukturen geprägt wird, weiterhin von den verschiedenen Zuschreibungen zu Ayurveda in einem „komplexen, diskursiven Netzwerk" (PATTATHU 2015: 322). Pattathu stellt diese Dynamiken letztendlich als Aushandlungsprozesse dar: So positionierten sich die Therapeuten und Therapeutinnen innerhalb des „biomedizinisch dominierten Feldes"[7] (PATTATHU 2015: 332) in einer Gemengelage von „Ganzheitsmedizin", spiritueller Praxis, Wellness und/oder Biomedizin.

Der Verfasser des vorliegenden Artikels führte Feldforschungen in verschiedenen deutschen Ayurveda-Einrichtungen mittels teilnehmender Beobachtung und qualitativer Interviews durch, ergänzt durch Internetrecherchen über die Selbstdarstellungen von Ayurveda-Einrichtungen (DOLLMANN 2021: 110–161). Online-Auftritte[8] von Ayurveda-Einrichtungen prägen die zugeschriebene „Ganzheitlichkeit" des Ayurveda unter Berücksichtigung von „Körper, Geist und Seele" vor. Es folgen Beispiele:

> Hier werden seit über 15 Jahren traditionelle Ayurvedakuren mit medizinischem Schwerpunkt im ganzheitlichen Sinne für Körper, Geist und Seele angeboten (SANTULAN-AUM KURZENTRUM 2010).

Sowohl die Seelen- als auch die Ganzheitssemantik werden zur Abgrenzung von der Schulmedizin häufig explizit angeführt, wie im Folgenden ersichtlich:

> Inwiefern unterscheidet sich eine Ayurveda Beratung von der modernen, westlichen Medizin? Nach der Auffassung des Ayurveda ist jede Form von Krankheit auf ein gestörtes Gleichgewicht der Elemente zurückzuführen. Im Ayurveda wird nicht ein einzelnes Symptom, sondern der Mensch als Ganzes behandelt. Geistige, seelisch orientierte und körperorientierte Therapieformen bilden die verschiedenen Bausteine eines fundierten Behandlungskonzeptes (AYURVAIDYA 2017).

Die Nähe von Ayurveda zu Spiritualität findet sich ebenfalls häufig in der Internetrecherche:[9]

> Der Ayurveda entspricht einigen Megatrends wie zum Beispiel der Individualisierung, dem Trend zu ganzheitlicher Gesundheit, Better Aging oder auch zu einer neuen Form der Spiritualisierung (BATRA 2010).

Auch in der Selbstverortung der Einrichtungen findet sich der Aspekt der Spiritualität:

> Ziel jeder individuell angepassten ayurvedischen Kur ist es, den Menschen mit all seinen Facetten zurück ins Gleichgewicht zu führen, damit er nicht nur körperlich gesunden, sondern auch seine spirituellen und geistigen positiven Anlagen entfalten kann (MAHARISHI AYURVEDA O. J.).

Ein erster Feldforschungsaufenthalt fand im Herbst 2015 in der Ayurveda-Abteilung der Habichtswald-Klinik Kassel statt, wobei der Verfasser als Arzt hospitieren konnte und somit einen Einblick in ayurvedische Untersuchungstechniken und Diagnostik bekommen konnte. Im Februar 2020 wurde die Feldforschung im Rosenberg Ayurveda Gesundheits- und Kurzentrum Birstein durchgeführt. Der Schwerpunkt lag hier auf dichter Beschreibung des Settings, teilnehmender Beobachtung und qualitativen Interviews mit Patientinnen und Patienten. In den Einrichtungen werden neben den ayurveda-typischen Anwendungen zahlreiche spirituelle Angebote, Meditations-Sitzungen und Yogastunden integriert. In Birstein wurde über Vorträge Ayurveda mit den Mythen hinduistischer Traditionen verbunden.

Dieser mentale Input ist verflochten mit dem sinnlichen Erleben der therapeutischen Angebote: Es kommt zu einer „sensorischen Wucht" (DOLLMANN 2021: 134) von multimodalen Sinneseindrücken: Fast in den gesamten Einrichtungen nimmt man den Geruch der mit Kräutern versetzten Ölen zu Massage wahr, ebenso den als exotisch empfundenen Geruch von Gewürzen der ayurvedischen Küche. Die Speisen – oft individuell auf die jeweiligen Ungleichgewichte der Patienten und Patientinnen bezogen – werden z. T. unter strengem Stillschweigen eingenommen, was die gustatorische Wahrnehmung optimiert. Haptische Eindrücke stehen im Vordergrund der Massagen mit Ölen oder geklärter Butter, teils durchgeführt durch zwei Therapierende simultan mit vier Händen. Akustische Impressionen werden in manchen Einrichtungen während Meditationen durch Om-Gesänge ausgelöst. Propriozeptoren führen zu oft ungewohnten Wahrnehmungen während der Yogaübungen. Die Optik wird in den Einrichtungen durch die Darstellung hinduistischer Gottheitsstatuen oder entsprechender Bilder in den Gängen und Behandlungsräumen geprägt. Die Summe der medialen Vorprägungen führt in Verbindung mit der sensorischen Wucht und perzeptiven Synthese des gesamten Settings zu der kognitiven und sinnlichen „Wahr"nehmung, zum Erleben einer „Ganzheitlichkeit", was sich in den Interviews bestätigen lässt. Von den Teilnehmenden werden viele Situationen sowohl während der therapeutischen Sitzungen als auch Wahrnehmungen außerhalb der Therapien als spirituell erlebt. Die Ayurvedatherapien werden meist komplementär zur Evidenzbasierten Medizin durchgeführt, aber in den Interviews wurde das Erleben der letzteren als fragmentierend betont. Im Folgenden werden kurze Ausschnitte aus den Interviews zu der Gemengelage „Ganzheitlichkeit" und „Spiritualität" angeführt, lediglich um die Erlebensebene an die zuvor historisch und kulturwissenschaftlich analysierten Befunde anzubinden. Auf die Frage, warum sie eine ayurvedische Behandlung aufsuche, antwortete eine Patientin:[10]

> [...] dass ich jetzt auch offen auf dem Hintergrund meiner christlichen Spiritualität ganzheitlichen Heilweisen, also dem Zusammenhang von geis-

tigen, seelischen und körperlichen Dingen, große Beachtung schenke (Patientin B1w, Birstein).

Folgende Aussage führt den Aspekt der Ganzheitlichkeit explizit zur Abgrenzung von der Schulmedizin an:

> [...] Beim Schulmediziner habe ich keine ganzheitliche Behandlung. Der fragt mich, was haben Sie für Beschwerden und drückt mir eine Tablette in die Hand. (Leicht lachend): so ganz krass mal ausgedrückt. [...] beim Ayurveda ist es so, da wird der ganze Mensch gesehen, und es wird mehr an der Ursache und auch an der Psyche gearbeitet, als es die Schulmedizin mir bietet. (Patientin B2w, Birstein).

Die ayurvedische Behandlung wird von den Patientinnen und Patienten zum Teil als eine spirituelle Erfahrung verstanden, zum Teil auch mit der hinduistischen Tradition verbunden:

> Also zum Beispiel wenn man über die Ganesha-Gottheit spricht, mit den großen Elefantenohren, der man seine Sorgen, alles anvertrauen kann, das ermutigt Menschen auch dazu, einen Weg zu finden, also andere Zugänge noch zu finden, sich von ihren Sorgen und Beschwerden zu lösen. Also das empfinde ich schon als eine spirituelle Atmosphäre (Patientin B1w, Birstein).

Auf die Frage, auf was sich die mit der Behandlung empfundene Spiritualität gründet, fand sich bei einer weiteren Patientin folgende Antwort:

> Dass ich Teil eines Ganzen bin [...] und dass ich in diesem Ganzen verbunden bin. Und zwar über Generationen bin ich verbunden. Ich bin nicht nur im Hier und Jetzt [...] Ich weiß zumindest, dass es da im spirituellen Sinne Seelen gibt, mit denen ich ganz eng verbunden bin (Patientin B6w, Birstein).

Spiritualität und eine Ganzheitserfahrung werden also individuell oft als zusammengehörig erlebt. Der Soziologe HUBERT KNOBLAUCH bezeichnet die CAM-Verfahren demgemäß auch als „Einfallstore des Spirituellen" (KNOBLAUCH 2010: 169). Auch der Kulturwissenschaftler FLORIAN JESERICH betont diesen Zusammenhang: Die Empfindung einer Fragmentierung in der Evidenzbasierten Medizin führe zur Suche nach einer „Ganzheitsmedizin", Patienten und Patien-

tinnen würden sich deswegen auf den „spirituellen Markt" (2010: 205–206) begeben, wo ein holistischer Heilungsbedarf gedeckt werde.

Resümee und Desiderata bezüglich einer „Integrativen Medizin"

Die akteursorientierte Wahrnehmung des gesamten multisensorischen Settings in den Ayurveda-Einrichtungen wurde zusammen mit den soziokulturellen, medialen Vorprägungen als Ausgangspunkt einer Ganzheitserfahrung analysiert, welche oft auch als spirituell erlebt wird. Zum Verständnis dieses Erlebens wurden nach der historischen Kontextualisierung kognitions- und neurowissenschaftliche Argumente mit Embodiment-Aspekten zusammengeführt. Das hier behandelte Problem der „Ganzheitlichkeit" lässt sich entlang dieser mehrperspektivischen, interdisziplinären Argumentationskette wie folgt zusammenfassen: Eine erstrebte „ganzheitliche" Erfassung des Menschen inklusive aller ihn beeinflussender Teile ist auf einer naturwissenschaftlich-empirisch fassbaren Ebene grundsätzlich nicht erreichbar. Ein „Ganzheitserleben" kann auf der phänomenologischen Ebene über qualitative Interviews erfasst werden: Die sinnliche Perzeption ist unser primärer Zugang zur Welt, und perzeptive Syntheseprozesse lassen uns eine kohärente Welt erleben (MERLEAU-PONTY 1964: 16; MOHR 2005: 621). Über diese Syntheseprozesse wird je nach soziokultureller und habitueller Vorprägung unsere „Wahr"nehmung konstruiert, die mehr oder weniger korreliert mit einer nicht vollständig zu verifizierenden Außenwelt. Non-Propositionalität des Körperwissens und Konstruktionsprozesse der Versprachlichung müssen in diesem Zusammenhang berücksichtigt werden (KOCH 2007: 279; KNOBLAUCH 2003: 32–33). Die Methodentriangulation in der vorliegenden Arbeit zeigt Synergien und plausibilisiert die Zusammenhänge zwischen Spiritualität und „Ganzheitserleben" im CAM-Bereich.

In dem beschriebenen Setting der Ayurveda-Einrichtungen lässt sich offensichtlich durch die oben beschriebene „sensorische Wucht" ein Kohärenzerleben erzeugen, das aus meiner Sicht und meiner medizinischen Erfahrung im Krankenhaus oder in einer Allgemeinpraxis schwierig zu erreichen scheint. Die gewonnenen Erkenntnisse im ayurvedischen Feld lassen sich auf Grund der unterschiedlichen sensorischen Voraussetzungen sicher auch nicht direkt auf andere CAM-Verfahren übertragen. Inwieweit dies eventuell möglich ist, wäre in weiteren Feldforschungen zu klären.

Als Konsequenz der vorliegenden Argumente wird folgende Hypothese aufgestellt: Es existiert ein Kontinuum zwischen einer Medizin, die als fragmentierend wahrgenommen wird, und medizinischen Verfahren, die „ganzheitlich" und evtl. auch spirituell wahrgenommen werden. In den Zuschreibungen von Patienten und Patientinnen sowie in manchen wissenschaftlichen Kommentaren steht die Schulmedizin auf Seiten der fragmentierenden Methoden (JESERICH 2010: 204; BÖKER 2003: A 24), auf der anderen Seite steht hier paradigmatisch Ayurveda mit der Zuschreibung der „Ganzheitlichkeit". In diesem postulierten Kontinuum ließen sich auch Methoden wie TCM, Bioresonanz, Osteopathie und andere CAM-Verfahren einordnen. Aus den hier vorgestellten Analysen lässt sich jedoch ableiten, dass die jeweilige Verortung auf dem angenommenen Kontinuum nicht beliebig sein kann. Sie ist sicher stark von der Persönlichkeit der Therapierenden und den habituellen Vorprägungen der Patientinnen und Patienten abhängig. Im Vordergrund steht jedoch das gesamte Setting mit den jeweils multimodal wahrnehmbaren Sinnesreizen.

Nach wechselseitiger Anerkennung der oben verorteten „Ganzheitlichkeit" auf der phänomenologischen Ebene könnte meines Erachtens zur Entgegenwirkung der möglichen Dichotomie von CAM und Evidenzbasierter Medizin die Erstellung eines Indikationen-Katalogs sinnvoll sein: Dazu könnte eine Liste von sogenannten funktionellen und reversiblen Erkrankungen (wie z.B. Migräne, Allergien, Schlafstörungen, Tinnitus etc.) erstellt werden, die nach einer Ausschlussdiagnostik primär und alternativ – also auch ausschließlich – einer CAM-Methode zugeführt werden können, wenn die Kranken dafür aufgeschlossen sind. Sehr früh könnten auch schon in der Anamneseerhebung die unterschiedlichen Erwartungshaltungen bezogen auf „Heilung" und/oder „Heil" berücksichtigt werden: Etymologisch geht das Wort „Heil" zurück auf das germanische *haila*, was „ganz" oder „unversehrt" bedeutet (AUFFARTH 2006: 203), auch heute wird das Wort „heil" umgangssprachlich oft für „ganz" verwendet. „Heil" stellt letztendlich die immanente Suche nach einer „Ganzheit" dar, die nicht nur mit der Suche nach den Ursachen von Leid, sondern auch der Suche nach transzendentem Sinn verbunden ist. Solche Ansätze finden sich zwar in der Evidenzbasierten Medizin schon jetzt im Bereich Spiritual Care in der Onkologie und im Hospizwesen. Die Berücksichtigung dieser Sinnsuche würde jedoch über onkologische Erkrankungen und Hospiz hinaus auch bei allen chronischen Erkrankungen den Zugang zu komplementären Therapien für evidenzbasierte Mediziner plausibilisieren. Selbstverständlich kann die Berücksichtigung der Sinnsuche in der hochspezialisierten Evidenzbasierten Medizin nur in einem sehr begrenzten Feld stattfinden: Gastroenterologen und Gastroenterologinnen beispielsweise müssen und sollen die Coloskopie so routiniert wie möglich durchführen. Dazu gehören neben der Ausbildung und technisch aktueller Einrichtung auch eine hohe Anzahl durchgeführter Untersuchungen, um diese Routine zu erhalten. Dort können Patientinnen und Patienten meist nur in Fragmenten wahrgenommen werden, ein Gespräch über Bedeutung und Sinn von Krankheiten wird wohl nicht stattfinden. Unter Berücksichtigung der in dieser Arbeit erfolgten Analysen ergibt sich jedoch ein Aufforderungscharakter an alle Schulmediziner- und medizinerinnen im allgemeinärztlichen oder hausärztlichen Bereich: Neben der zeitintensiveren Anamneseerhebung – betreffend oben erwähnter Erwartungshaltungen – sollte aus meiner Argumentation heraus dem sinnlich wahrnehmbaren Setting einer Praxis mehr Aufmerksamkeit gewidmet werden. Das beginnt schon mit der unmittelbaren Zuwendung durch Blick und Körperhaltung von Seiten der medizinischen Fachangestellten, wenn ein hilfesuchender Mensch die Praxis betritt. Bilder aus dem Bereich Kunst oder Natur, vielleicht verbunden mit anregenden schriftlichen Informationen, beeinflussen die emotionale Wahrnehmung vermutlich positiver als Plakate und Hinweise auf Leistungen, die nicht von der Krankenkasse bezahlt werden können. Unangenehme Gerüche z.B. nach Desinfektionsmitteln oder Therapiegeräusche sollten in Wartebereichen nicht wahrnehmbar sein. Als Ärztinnen und Ärzte müssten wir darüber hinaus in vielen Situationen neben der technisch-apparativen Diagnostik, deren wir uns bedienen dürfen, wieder vermehrt auf die Bedeutung einer intensiven körperlichen Untersuchung achten, die Patientinnen und Patienten „berühren", um auf Augenhöhe unsere Ansprüche wechselseitig wieder mehr zu „begreifen". Die Konsultationsgespräche sollten zudem ihre Asymmetrie verlieren, eine entsprechend offenere Gesprächsführung kann zu besseren Therapieergebnissen führen (KESSLER, EISENMANN, OBERZAUCHER, FORSTER, STECKHAN, MEIER, STAPELFELDT, MICHALSEN, & JEITLER 2017: 61–65). Die zunehmende Inanspruchnahme von CAM verweist ja auf ebendiese Defizite in der Ausübung und Selbstpräsentation der Evidenzbasierten Medizin in Hausarztpraxen und Krankenhäusern (JESERICH 2010: 204; BÖKER 2003: A 24–27).

Das Ziel müsste m. E. eine Integrative Medizin ohne gegenseitige Ausschlussdiskurse sein. Dem Verfasser ist aus jahrzehntelanger Erfahrung in allgemeinärztlicher internistischer Praxis das Problem der Zeit und der Vergütung bekannt, aber die Vergegenwärtigung der Problematik ist Grundvoraussetzung berufspolitischer Lösungsstrategien.

Anmerkungen

1 Der Begriff „anthropologisch" bezieht sich in dieser Arbeit schwerpunktmäßig auf die Philosophische Anthropologie und die Leibesphänomenologie i. S. von Maurice Merleau-Ponty. Einen Überblick hierzu bieten FISCHER 2009 und GROSSHEIM & THIES 2009.
2 Die Begriffe „Religion" und „Spiritualität" sind europäischen Ursprungs. In der frühen Geschichte hinduistischer und buddhistischer Traditionen lässt sich somit auch keine Abgrenzung zu „Philosophie" vornehmen, das Zeichen „/" will dies verdeutlichen. Seit der kolonialen Verflechtungsgeschichte spätestens ab dem 19. Jahrhundert ist der Begriff „Religion" jedoch nicht mehr als eine westliche Spezifität zu fassen (BERGUNDER 2011: 50–55). Hinduistische und buddhistische Traditionen werden in der Religionswissenschaft als „Religion" untersucht.
3 Kulturwissenschaftlich besteht Konsens, dass es „den Hinduismus" nicht gibt, sondern zahlreiche hinduistische Traditionen. Vivekananda stellte seine Interpretation des advaita vedanta 1893 jedoch als „Hinduismus" dar.
4 Es gibt im Zusammenhang „ganzheitlicher" Heilung und Spiritualität auch Einfluss nehmende europäische

Persönlichkeiten in der Geschichte. Auch die christliche Mystikerin und Heilkundige Hildegard von Bingen (1098–1179) sah Mensch und Kosmos als Einheit (PERNOUD 1996: 97). Ihre Popularität außerhalb von Fachkreisen stieg jedoch enorm erst in den letzten Jahrzehnten. Das „[...] bedeutendste und eindrucksvollste Werk über Hildegard von Bingen [...]" (PERNOUD 1996: 7) erschien 1982, also auch erst in der zweiten Hälfte des 20. Jahrhunderts zeitgleich mit der Popularisierung von CAM-Verfahren.
5 Bei Zitaten vor der Rechtschreibreform wird auf ein (sic!) verzichtet.
6 Eine Übersicht zu diesen Transformationen findet sich neben SMITH & WUJASTYK 2008 beispielsweise bei KOCH 2005, LANGFORD 2002 und ZYSK 2001.
7 Der Begriff „Biomedizin" wird überwiegend in der Anthropologie verwendet und darf hier synonym mit „Evidenzbasierter Medizin" verstanden werden.
8 Um subjektive Vorauswahlen zu vermeiden, wurden auf dem PC vor der Recherche sämtliche Cookies und der Internetverlauf gelöscht und nur die ersten zehn Einträge zu „Ayurveda-Einrichtungen" in der Google-Suche verwertet.
9 Die Homepage *Journal für ein gesünderes Leben* fand sich ebenfalls unter den ersten zehn Einträgen der unter Anmerkung 8 gefundenen Seiten.
10 Die angeführten Interviewauszüge wurden sprachlich geglättet. Die vollständigen Transkriptionen der Interviews mit nur leichter Sprachglättung finden sich bei DOLLMANN 2021: 229–294.

Literatur

AMMERMAN, NANCY TATOM 2013. Spiritual But Not Religious? Beyond Binary Choices in the Study of Religion. *Journal for the Scientific Study of Religion* 52, 2: 258–278.
AUFFARTH, CHRISTOPH 2006. Heil/Leid. In AUFFARTH, CHRISTOPH; KIPPENBERG, HANS & MICHAELS, AXEL (eds) *Wörterbuch der Religionen*. Stuttgart: Kröner: 203–205.
AYURVAIDYA 2017. Über uns. https://www.ayurvaidya.de/ueber-uns [06.03.2022].
BATRA, DAVID 2010. Ayurveda in Deutschland. *Ayurveda Journal für ein gesünderes Leben* 28, 4. https://www.ayurveda-journal.de/ayurveda-deutschen-gesundheitseinrichtungen/ [06.03.2020].
BERGUNDER 2011. Was ist Religion? Kulturwissenschaftliche Überlegungen zum Gegenstand der Religionswissenschaft. *Zeitschrift für Religionswissenschaft* 19, 1/2: 3–55.
BERGUNDER, MICHAEL 2012. Indischer Swami und deutscher Professor ‚Religion' jenseits des Eurozentrismus. In STAUSBERG, MICHAEL (ed) *Religionswissenschaft*. Berlin, Boston: de Gruyter: 95–07.
BERGUNDER, MICHAEL 2016. „Religion" and „Science" within a Global Religious History. *Aries* 16: 86–141.
BERGUNDER, MICHAEL 2020. Umkämpfte Historisierung. Die Zwillingsgeburt von „Religion" und „Esoterik" in der zweiten Hälfte des 19. Jahrhunderts und das Programm einer globalen Religionsgeschichte. In KLAUS HOCK (ed) *Wissen um Religion: Erkenntnis – Interesse Epistemologie und Epis-*

teme in Religionswissenschaft und Interkultureller Theologie. Leipzig: Evangelische Verlagsanstalt: 47–131.

BOCHINGER, CHRISTOPH 1995. „New Age"und moderne Religion. Religionswissenschaftliche Analysen. Gütersloh: Kaiser [orig. 1994].

BÖKER, WOLFGANG 2003. Der fragmentierte Patient. Deutsches Ärzteblatt 1, 2: A 24–A 27.

CAPRA, FRITJOF 1985. Vorwort. In MILZ, HELMUT Ganzheitliche Medizin. Neue Wege zur Gesundheit. Mit einem Vorwort von Fritjof Capra. Königstein/Ts.: Athenäum: 9–14.

CHOPRA, ANANDA S. 2012: Pancakarma-Therapie im Ayurveda: Eine gute Therapie für Gesunde und Kranke. Erfahrungsheilkunde 61: 10–16.

CSORDAS, THOMAS J. 1990. Embodiment as a Paradigm for Anthropology. Ethos 18, 1: 5–47.

DILGER, HANSJÖRG & SCHNEPF, MAX 2020. Alternative Gesundheitsvorstellungen und -praktiken in der deutschen Therapielandschaft: Bericht zur Literaturrecherche „Vielfalt im Gesundheitswesen" im Auftrag der Robert Bosch Stiftung GmbH. https://refubium.fu-berlin.de/bitstream/handle/fub188/26768/Bericht%20BoschStiftung%20Final.pdf?sequence=1&isAllowed=y [30.11.2022].

DOLLMANN, JÜRGEN W. 2021. Spirituelle Diskurse und Performanzen in deutschen Ayurveda-Einrichtungen. Transdisziplinäre, integrative Analyse eines ,ganzheitlichen' Therapieverfahrens. Inauguraldissertation. Heidelberg: Universität Heidelberg.

EISENMANN, CLEMENS; KLEIN, CONSTANTIN; SWHAJOR-BIESEMANN, ANNE; DREXELIUS, UWE; KELLER, BARBARA & STREIB, HEINZ 2016. Dimensions of „Spirituality". The Semantics of Subjective Definitions. In STREIB, HEINZ & HOOD, RALPH W. (eds) Semantics and Psychology of Spirituality. A Cross-Cultural Analysis. Cham, Heidelberg: Springer: 125–151.

ERASMUS DESIDERIUS 2008. Encomium Artis Medicae. Lob der Heilkunst, Lateinisch/Deutsch, BERGDOLT, KLAUS (ed) (Übers.), Heidelberg: Manutius.

FIGL, JOHANN 2003. Handbuch Religionswissenschaft. Innsbruck: Tyrolia.

FISCHER, JOACHIM 2009. Philosophische Anthropologie. In BOHLKEN, EIKE & THIES, CHRISTIAN (eds) Handbuch Anthropologie. Der Mensch zwischen Natur, Kultur und Technik. Weimar: Metzler: 216–224.

FRASS, MICHAEL; STRASSL, ROBERT PAUL; FRIEHS, HELMUT; MÜLLNER, MICHAEL; KUNDI, MICHAEL & KAYE, ALAN D. 2012. Use and Acceptance of Complementary and Alternative Medicine Among the General Population and Medical Personnel: A Systematic Review. The Ochsner Journal 12, 1: 45–56.

GROSSHEIM, MICHAEL & THIES, CHRISTIAN 2009. Phänomenologie. In BOHLKEN, EIKE & THIES, CHRISTIAN (eds) Handbuch Anthropologie. Der Mensch zwischen Natur, Kultur und Technik. Weimar: Metzler: 208–16.

HAHNEMANN, SAMUEL 1999. Organon der Heilkunst. Aude sapere. Stuttgart: Karl F. Haug [auf der Grundlage der 1992 vom Herausgeber bearbeiteten textkritischen Ausgabe des Manuskriptes Hahnemanns von 1842].

HANEGRAAFF, WOUTER J. 1996. New Age Religion and Western Culture. Esotericism in the Mirror of Secular Thought. Leiden: Brill.

HANEGRAAFF, WOUTER J. 2007. New Age Movement and Western Esotericism. In KEMP, DAREN & LEWIS, JAMES R. (eds) Handbook of New Age. Leiden: Brill: 25–50.

HEELAS, PAUL & WOODHEAD, LINDA 2005. The Spiritual Revolution. Why Religion is Giving Way to Spirituality. Oxford: Blackwell.

HERO, MARKUS 2009. Das Prinzip „Access". Zur institutionellen Infrastruktur zeitgenössischer Spiritualität. Zeitschrift für Religionswissenschaft 17: 189–211.

HÖLLINGER, FRANZ & TRIPOLD, THOMAS 2012. Ganzheitliches Leben. Das holistische Milieu zwischen neuer Spiritualität und postmoderner Wellness-Kultur, Bielefeld: transcript.

HOUTMAN, DICK & AUPERS, STEF 2009. The spiritual revolution and the New Age gender puzzle: The sacralisation of the self in late modernity (1980–2000). Journal for the Scientific Study of Religion. 46, 3: 305–320.

JÄCKLE, RENATE 1985. Gegen den Mythos Ganzheitliche Medizin. Hamburg: Konkret Literatur.

JESERICH, FLORIAN 2010. Spirituelle/religiöse Weltanschauungen als Herausforderung für unser Gesundheitswesen. Am Beispiel der Homöopathie. In BECKER, RAYMOND (ed) „Neue" Wege in der Medizin. Alternativmedizin – Fluch oder Segen? Heidelberg: Winter: 203–227.

JÜTTE, ROBERT 1996. Geschichte der Alternativen Medizin. Von der Volksmedizin zu den unkonventionellen Therapien von heute. München: C. H. Beck.

JÜTTE, ROBERT 2017. Medizinischer Pluralismus. Was wir aus der Geschichte lernen können. Festansprache zur Eröffnung des LMHI World Congress Leipzig 2017 am 14.06.2017. Allgemeine Homöopathische Zeitung. 262, 6: 4–9.

KAISER, JOCHEN 2018. Wahrnehmung. In DEINZER; RENATE & VON DEM KNESEBECK, OLAF (eds) Online Lehrbuch der Medizinischen Psychologie und Medizinischen Soziologie. https://books.publisso.de/en/publisso_gold/publishing/books/overview/46/85 [12.01.2021].

KESSLER, CHRISTIAN; WISCHNEWSKY, MANFRED; MICHALSEN, ANDREAS & EISENMANN, CLEMENS & MELZER, JÖRG 2013. Ayurveda. Between Religion, Spirituality, and Medicine. Evidence-Based Complementary and Alternative Medicine. https://doi.org/10.1155/2013/952432 [01.12.2022].

KESSLER, CHRISTIAN; EISENMANN, CLEMENS; OBERZAUCHER, FRANK; FORSTER, MARTIN; STECKHAN, NICO; MEIER, LARISSA; STAPELFELDT, ELMAR; MICHALSEN, ANDREAS & JEITLER, MICHAEL 2017. Ayurvedic versus conventional dietary and lifestyle counseling for mothers with burnout-syndrome. A randomized controlled pilot study including a qualitative evaluation. Complementary Therapies in Medicine 34: 57–65.

KING, RICHARD 1999. Orientalism and Religion. Postcolonial theory, India and the mystic „East". London, New York: Routledge.

KING, RICHARD 2007. Mysticism and Spirituality. In HINNELLS, JOHN R. (ed) The Routledge Companion to the Study of Religion. London, New York: Routledge: 306–322.

KNOBLAUCH, HUBERT 2003. *Qualitative Religionsforschung. Religionsethnographie in der eigenen Gesellschaft.* Paderborn, München, Wien, Zürich: Schöningh.

KNOBLAUCH, HUBERT 2010. Vom New Age zur populären Spiritualität. In LÜDDECKENS, DOROTHEA & WALTHERT, RAFAEL (eds) *Fluide Religion. Neue religiöse Bewegungen im Wandel. Theoretische und empirische Systematisierungen.* Bielefeld: Transcript: 149–174.

KOCH, ANNE 2005. Spiritualisierung eines Heilwissens im lokalen religiösen Feld? Zur Formierung deutscher Ayurveden. *Zeitschrift für Religionswissenschaft* 13, 1: 21–44.

KOCH, ANNE 2006. Wie Medizin und Heilsein wieder verwischen. Ethische Plausibilisierungsmuster des Ayurveda im Westen. *Zeitschrift für Medizinische Ethik* 52: 169–182.

KOCH, ANNE 2007. *Körperwissen. Grundlegung einer Religionsaisthetik.* Habilitationsschrift. Ludwig-Maximilians-Universität München: München.

LANGFORD, JEAN M. 2002. *fluent bodies. Ayurvedic Remedies for Postcolonial Imbalance.* Durham, London: Duke University Press.

LÜDDECKENS, DOROTHEA 2012. Religion und Medizin in der europäischen Moderne. In STAUSBERG, MICHAEL (ed) *Religionswissenschaft.* Berlin/Boston: de Gruyter: 283–297.

MAHARISHI AYURVEDA o. J. Ayurveda Kur in Deutschland. Individuell & authentisch. https://www.ayurveda-badems.de/ayurveda-kuren/ [24.04.2021].

MERLEAU-PONTY, MAURICE 1964. The Primacy of Perception. In MERLEAU-PONTY, MAURICE *The Primacy of Perception. And Other Essays on Phenomenological Psychology, the Philosophy of Art, History and Politics.* Evanston: Northwestern University Press: 12–42.

MOHN, JÜRGEN 2007. Körperkonzepte in der Religionswissenschaft und der Religionsgeschichte. In AUS DER AU, CHRISTINA & PLÜSS, DAVID (eds) *Körper – Kulte. Wahrnehmung von Leiblichkeit in Theologie, Religions- und Kulturwissenschaften.* Zürich: Theologischer Verlag Zürich: 47–73.

MOHR, HUBERT 2005. Wahrnehmung/Sinnessystem. In AUFFARTH, CHRISTOPH; BERNARD, JUTTA & MOHR, HUBERT (eds) *Metzler Lexikon Religion. Gegenwart – Alltag – Medien.* Stuttgart/Weimar: Metzler: 620–633.

O'REGAN, J. KELVIN & NOÉ, ALVA 2013. Ein sensomotorischer Ansatz des Sehens und des visuellen Bewusstseins. In FINGERHUT, JOERG; HUFENDIEK, REBEKKA & WILD, MARKUS (eds) *Philosophie der Verkörperung. Grundlagentexte zu einer aktuellen Debatte.* Berlin: Suhrkamp: 328–378.

PATTATHU, ANTONY G. 2015. Ayurveda als Aushandlungsort religiöser Verkörperung? Eine Fallstudie aus Deutschland. In KLINKHAMMER, GRITT & TOLKSDORF, EVA (eds) *Somatisierung des Religiösen. Empirische Studien zum rezenten religiösen Heilungs- und Therapiemarkt.* Bremen: Universität Bremen: 301–337.

PERNOUD RÉGINE 1996. *Hildegard von Bingen. Ihre Welt – Ihr Wirken – Ihre Vision.* Freiburg im Breisgau: Herder.

SACKETT, DAVID L. et al. 1996. Evidence based medicine. What it is and what it isn't. *British Medical Journal* 12: 71–72.

SANTULAN-AUM KURZENTRUM 2010. AUM-Kurzentrum – der Pionier für Ayurvedakuren feiert sein 15 Jähriges Bestehen in Deutschland. https://ayurvedakuren.com/aum-kurzentrum-15-jahre/ [06.03.2020].

SMITH, FREDERIK & WUJASTYK, DAGMAR 2008. Introduction. In WUJASTYK, DAGMAR & SMITH, FREDERIK M. (eds) *Modern and Global Ayurveda. Pluralism and Paradigms.* Albany: State Univ. of New York Press: 1–28.

VIVEKANANDA, SWAMI 1958a. *The Complete Works of Swami Vivekananda. Mayavati Memorial Edition III.* Advaita Ashrama: Calcutta.

VIVEKANANDA, SWAMI 1958b. *The Complete Works of Swami Vivekananda. Mayavati Memorial Edition II.* Advaita Ashrama: Calcutta.

WHO (ed) 2019. The WHO Global Report on Traditional and Complementary Medicine. https://apps.who.int/iris/bitstream/handle/10665/312342/9789241515436-eng.pdf?sequence=1&isAllowed=y [22.01.2021].

ZINSER, HARTMUT 2005. Magie und Medizin. Frobenius-Vorlesung 2004. *Paideuma* 51: 23–40.

ZYSK, KENNETH GREGORY 2001. New Age Ayurveda or What Happens to Indian Medi-cine. When it Comes to America. *Traditional South Asian Medicine* 6: 10–26.

Manuskript erhalten: 15.03.2022
Manuskript angenommen: 22.12.2022

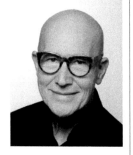

JÜRGEN W. DOLLMANN Dr. phil. Dr. med., Studium der Humanmedizin an der Universität Tübingen als Stipendiat der Studienstiftung des Deutschen Volkes, Promotion 1978. Weiterbildung zur Anerkennung als Internist. Insgesamt 34 Jahre ärztliche Tätigkeit in Krankenhaus und Praxis. Ab 2013 Studium der Religionswissenschaft an der Universität Heidelberg. 2021 Promotion, seit 2018 Lehrbeauftragter am Institut für Religionswissenschaft der Universität Heidelberg mit den Schwerpunkten Embodiment-Theorien, Theorien des verkörperten Geistes und dem Grenzbereich zwischen Religion und Medizin. Seit 2017 Mitglied im Arbeitskreis „Religion und Medizin" der Deutschen Vereinigung für Religionswissenschaft.

Universität Heidelberg, Institut für Religionswissenschaft
Fischmarkt 2, 69117 Heidelberg
juergen.dollmann@zegk.uni-heidelberg.de

FORUM
FORUM

Researching Pandemics from Below

An Interview with the Medical Historian Frédéric Vagneron
by Janina Kehr & Ehler Voss

Interview recorded on January 25, 2021
Transcription by Daria Ledergerber

Janina Kehr & Ehler Voss As a historian of medicine and science, you have been working for a decade on the science and epidemiology of the 1918 flu in France, also known as the Spanish Flu. During your extensive archival research across the country, you have become increasingly interested in a historiographical approach that one could term "from below". Historians like Arlette Farge (2019) and Michel Foucault have advocated this approach, for example in Foucault's famous text "La vie des homes infâmes" (1977). One aim of this approach was to give visibility to the voices of those who are rarely heard in official, institutional accounts. To what degree is this approach relevant for the Spanish flu? And where do you see its originality?

Frédéric Vagneron I think I need to start with the historiography of the Spanish flu: it bears the mark of an American historian, Alfred Crosby, who wrote the book "Epidemic and peace" in 1976, and it then became "the forgotten pandemic" ten years later when it was republished during the HIV/AIDS pandemic (Crosby 1976, 1989). This book was innovative in many ways: it framed the story of the Spanish flu pandemic in an American context as a "forgotten" event. This narrative has been the leading one for a long time for the scholars working on the 1918 pandemic.

It's a very provocative way to frame the story of the Spanish flu, considering the huge death toll of the 1918 flu in the US and elsewhere: you may know that the last estimate of the death toll during the Spanish flu is between 50 and 100 million people (Johnson & Mueller 2002). Hence the big enigma: how is it possible to have a forgotten pandemic and at the same time something that was so deadly? That was my starting point as a scholar: was it forgotten? In what ways was it

forgotten? Is it a question of memory? Is it a question of the event as a process? Is it the official and national sources used by historians and the questions they brought to interrogate them? A lot of different questions!

In different national contexts, historians have been working with this US-centric narrative. But other historical narratives are also crucial to understand how the Spanish flu has been experienced.

In Europe for instance, the prominent narrative was that of the Great War, the tremendous human loss and its social consequences. In France, 1.4 million people died during the Great War: the Spanish flu broke out only at the end of the war and represents only a fraction of the population loss during this time of crisis. The pandemic started during the spring of 1918 and ended during the negotiations leading to the Treaty of Versailles in 1919. From the statistics, it is difficult to say precisely how many people died from the flu pandemic in France, but roughly 250,000. In France and in Europe, the Great War has been a leading field in historiography, which made it more difficult to study the Spanish flu event per se, while placing it in the specific context of the war.

Working on the Spanish flu "from below" means trying to access how the population experienced the pandemic and its many temporalities and social traces in societies profoundly affected by the war. What are the temporalities of the pandemic? It sounds like an easy question! But it is much more complex than what you might think. You need to question the temporalities of an epidemic proposed by Charles Rosenberg (Rosenberg 1989). The story of epidemics as dramaturgic forms (with a beginning, a peak, and an end) does not fit so well when you are working on the Spanish flu in 1918 (and probably even less in the face of a disease like Covid, which is caused by different strains with various temporalities of propagation and epidemiological signatures). The beginning of the pandemic remained "silent" during the spring of 1918, the peak of the autumn wave was blurred by the last military offensives and the armistice, and the end of the pandemic stayed rather unnoticed if you look at the main official archives ...

What was the experience of the people not only through the lenses of the state, science, and medicine? When you work in the archives, you collect new material and start to build a new understanding of the Spanish influenza that connects small insights gathered in different archival stocks. Some come from soldiers, some from families. The war itself created its specific archives: for instance, the correspondence between the soldiers on the front and their families. This type of archives is interesting because, despite the military censorship, you access other layers of experience: what is happening to the soldiers at the front, how they tell their relatives or what they don't say about the epidemic, what they actually know about the epidemic elsewhere in the country, and how they worry about what is happening on the home front.

From that starting point, "the forgotten pandemic" narrative is challenged by various local archival traces. This alternative account of the pandemic is important, because it makes you think about the variety of experiences from one place to the other, from one community or social group to the other, from one individual to another. In 1918, the population and the authorities had some understanding that the pandemic was international in its propagation, but that does not mean that its consequences are similar everywhere.

It sounds obvious in the light of the Covid-19 pandemic, but it is a challenge to document a century-old event that now is remembered as a global scourge. What becomes clear when you collect the sources is that the experience of the epidemic, even in one country, is really fragmented both in temporalities and geographically. Variability becomes an essential concept; it describes the variety of the symptoms, of the experiences, and the tremendous challenge for the medical profession, scientists, and states.

Janina Kehr & Ehler Voss Let's stick with the question of fragmentation and regional and national variability, also to get a better idea of how you work as a medical historian. You have worked on France in particular. How was the 1918 flu archived there? You have already mentioned military archives, as well as communications between soldiers at the front and their homes. So what were your different archival sources, where did you find them?

Frédéric Vagneron The main archival places where you find some information about the influenza pandemic are, of course, the public archives. But in France in 1918, there is no ministry of Health or Public Hygiene. The main department of health belongs to the "Home Office" (*Ministère de l'Intérieur*). And most of its archives burned during World War Two ... Furthermore, the Great War had a huge impact on the way the population's health is handled. The military medical archives (*archives du service de santé militaire*) are crucial for understanding how the pandemic was dealt with in 1918. Most of the men were in the army and the incorporation of civilian doctors in military service had a profound impact on the management of health in the civilian population. But these military archives had no detailed catalogue before the first decade of the 21st century. These archives tell you a story of the epidemic in the military, but you also gain some insight about what was going on in the countryside and cities far away from the battlefield, as military doctors were sent to the civilian population in emergencies.

Local archives are then the bulk of the sources. During my PhD, I went to many towns in France, around 25 municipal archival settings, to look at both municipal and departmental sources. The *department archive* provides you with information not only on the bigger cities, but also on villages and the countryside. That's almost the only way to know what is going on, on this local scale.

But the sources there are very heterogeneous. I went to Brest in Brittany, for instance, because the influenza epidemic was reported first in the American troops crossing the Atlantic during Spring 1918: but you have no mention of influenza in the archives before late August 1918. Then I went to Paris, of course, Lyon, Montpellier,

Tours, Grenoble, etc. I went to Marseille; surprisingly, there was almost nothing about the flu even during the peak of the pandemic in September-November 1918. Public health officials were still talking about the cholera of the 19th century and the risk of epidemics coming from the Mediterranean Sea. In the beginning of 1919, there was also a minor typhus epidemic, on which all public attention focused, because such an epidemic would be a major blow to public health after the war. You know at the same time that the influenza pandemic was in its third wave in the country: but in the archives, you have almost nothing about influenza.

So, at first, I was trying to collect all the traces that I could find, starting with the public health institutions, but more and more I found documents showing a silent tide of the pandemic that needed additional inquiry. For my research, a way to focus more on this approach of the "history from below" was to look at funeral services.

Janina Kehr & Ehler Voss Why the archives of funeral services?

Frédéric Vagneron Why did I use this approach to work on influenza? It's because influenza was and still is a difficult disease for doctors to name because of its many complications and its blurry clinical picture. When practitioners or civil registrars wrote the cause of death on the death certificates, it was sometimes influenza, but most of the time it was other diseases: bronchial pneumonia, pneumonia, etc. Of course, this raises questions about the reliability of the statistics. But whatever the cause of death is—if influenza is written on the death certificate or if it is something else—authorities and families had to deal with the dead bodies. So how did they manage to deal with these dead bodies in this time of crisis?

Here I was building on an important body of literature available about different recent health crises, such as the big heat waves in Chicago in 1995 and in France in 2003. Hurricane Katrina was also something that was really interesting to me, because you have this "natural" event revealing social inequalities. The question of the management of dead bodies, hidden behind the mortality figures or medical controversies, is fascinating (LAQUEUR 2015). It brings up the ways

the community faces an event that might be invisible elsewhere in the sources and the potential rupture that the health crisis brings in public opinion when the deceased are not treated with the dignity that corresponds to the norms of the time. It also brings up the memory of past pandemic events and "the plague narrative" associated with mass graves: that's something that came back again during Covid in New York, in Manaus, Brazil, and in France (Rungis, a Paris suburban area, became a temporary place to store coffins and bodies at the end of March 2020 because of the increase in mortality in the Paris area). So, this line of research became a way to systematize my research on this other narrative, going beyond the hypothesis of the forgotten pandemic.

I compared the management of corpses in Paris and in Grenoble in 1918. Grenoble experienced a major crisis. The local administration had outsourced funeral activities to a private company: they were unable to deal with the huge number of dead bodies in October. There were public investigations following this crisis, and the socialist press accused the municipality of mismanagement.

In contrast, in the archives in Paris, I found much information about the management of dead bodies in 1918, which was striking in comparison with the lack of documents in the public health boxes. That's the pleasure of the historian: I always think that there is a mine of information somewhere in the archives and I just need to find the right key to order the right box. If it is not the one labeled "Influenza pandemic", then it's just that you have to order something else. What you need here is the right question: and for me it was the role if the funeral service in the crisis process. I found that the organization of Parisian funeral services made it possible to continue acting to cope with the sudden increase in burials. But you need to relocate what happened in 1918 in the situation of the service the previous years. Paris had built its own municipal service after a law in 1904 and used a big building in the North of Paris, created at the end of the 19th century, and employed more than 1,000 people to organize the funeral services. They called it "l'usine de la mort"—the "death factory"—and in this huge building, people sawed wood for and assembled the coffins, there were tailors, there were the grooms and drivers of horse-drawn carriages … At the end of October 1918, the Parisian funeral services carried out nearly 500 burials daily. Thanks to the hard work of hundreds of employees, the epidemic in Paris did not cause a scandal like the one that took place at the same time in Grenoble.

These two cases allow us to contrast certain decisive factors. The political choice to delegate direct responsibility for the management of the dead to the municipalities: this was the case in Paris in the form of a municipal funeral service under the direction of the Prefecture of the Seine, which most certainly made it possible to deal with the mortality crisis. In contrast, the Grenoble funeral service, subcontracted to a private firm, was unable to adapt as quickly to the influx of victims, leading to a radical questioning of the municipal authorities, who were deemed responsible for the dramatic situation.

This work shows that the capacity to manage a situation of extraordinary mortality rates also rests on previous transformations in how bodies were buried: based on the archive material, I can emphasize the role of the new cemeteries created on the outskirts of Paris, which made it possible to "absorb" the quantity of corpses, often of people belonging to the least privileged classes of the population. Many new cemeteries were located extramurally, outside of Paris, but they belonged to the municipality. The famous Père Lachaise cemeteries and the cemeteries Montmartre and Montparnasse were the big ones in the 19th century. But they were crowded. They created new ones in Pantin, Evry, etc. at the end of the 19th century. The lower social classes were buried in these cemeteries outside of the city. The rich people would still have some vaults in the cemeteries in Paris. Rich families would still have the traditional gathering of people coming to the funeral service during the pandemic in 1918. But most of the population was burying its dead with much less visibility in the big cemeteries outside Paris. One local politician in Clichy, for instance, tells in his Great War diary, that he is attending the funeral of his niece in October 1918. He describes this event in a very shadowy and lugubrious tone. His narrative depicts how the service works to bring the coffin to Pantin.

Overall, in Paris, the invisibilization of death in the time of the epidemic is the result of the public management's success: the extreme flow of mortality was mitigated thanks to an extraordinary adaptation to the epidemic challenge and to a differentiated spatial treatment of the dead according to their income. Maintaining an industrial, but decent management of death in the autumn of 1918 avoided the political scandal that was rampant in Grenoble at the same time. But it was at the cost of a drastic restriction of the funeral rite and of a generalized anonymity, breaking with the fast that distinguished previously individual funerals and with the emerging celebration of the lost heroes of the war (cp. VAGNERON 2022).

Janina Kehr & Ehler Voss   What material would you like to be available for Covid-19 historians in the future?

Frédéric Vagneron   That is a difficult question, because what you want to document is the variability of the disease and of the experience of the sickness: not only telling the story of people who died from influenza or Covid—but also the story of the people who got sick (including with this debated category of Long Covid) and those who had no direct contact with the disease.

One thing that is really important in the Covid pandemic is the role of the hospital system. The lockdown policies in France, for instance, were related to the fear of having a big wave overwhelming the hospital system. The challenge was to avoid forcing professionals in the hospital to implement triage between two different patients diagnosed with Covid or something else. The lockdown policies were really related to the hospital infrastructure. It is really different from one country to the other. In general, I find it enlightening to think about how hospitals in the most developed countries encountered problems of lack of beds, staff, or drugs—shortages that have historically been associated with the most disadvantaged countries in the world.

On a more pragmatic and dramatic level, there is an obstacle to telling the story of people dying in the hospital. We read in the news many articles about people who entered the hospitals with a cough or short of breath and who didn't feel so bad at the beginning of their sickness. Many of them stayed for several weeks in intensive care without their families and eventually died. How do you tell this story? How can you relate their experience and the experiences of their families? More generally, the experience of the health care professionals is also at stake, the nurses and doctors, etc.: all the grieving process becomes really difficult to document and to interpret. A year and a half later, with the vaccination campaigns now implemented and the political concerns about the return to normalcy (fueled by the health passport device), this aspect of emergency is already difficult to bring back.

Janina Kehr & Ehler Voss In our Curare Corona Diaries project, we collected diaries and intended to record the everyday aspects of the Covid-19 pandemic in different locations, also in anticipation of potential future historical research. As a historian of the present, how would you research this archive?

Frédéric Vagneron You first need to know who the people are whom you are investigating. You cannot compare one diary and the other just like that because of Covid-19. Covid-19 is a really fragmented experience … even for the doctors. The pediatrician looks at something, the dermatologist finds new symptoms, the internist looks at something else … and to me, the danger is in recreating an artificial common experience under the label Covid-19.

It is crucial to collect these diaries with all the methodological precautions. It's well documented in sociology and anthropology: people are going to answer your questions; the interview setting is not a natural discussion, but an artifact that carries many biases. Even if the person never thought about the question you ask, you will get an answer. It also means that you need to design your research in such a way as to find people who, for many reasons, did not care about Covid and its experience, to elucidate a sort of "zero" in the statistics. You need these other testimonies to control that you are not creating the information and the interpretation that you originally wanted. The list of questions that you use will somehow artificially connect people. Then I think it is interesting to enrich the analysis and your corpus with other documents to recreate the environment that is specific to each individual.

Janina Kehr & Ehler Voss Your methodological caution ties in well with our following question. The Covid-19 pandemic is being portrayed as a profound transformation of life for everybody, and yet, not everybody experiences or is impacted by the pandemic in the same way. Covid-19 is without doubt a global crisis in multiple ways, but many voices also question this crisis narrative, this narrative of exception. What was it like in 1918? How did the 1918 flu affect people differently? With 100 years of hindsight, what can be said about the tension between the crisis, the state of emergency, and the continuation of everyday life in 1918?

Frédéric Vagneron There are really interesting studies that have been done, mainly in North America, and I really recommend a look at the work of ESYLLT JONES (2007). She worked on the Spanish flu in Winnipeg, Canada, and she explains how people dealt with having a father who died, what kind of solidarity emerged from this situation, and how the pandemic gave more visibility to women in the public sphere. The epidemic revealed the burden of inequalities in Canadian society, for instance in status and ethnicity. NANCY BRISTOW (2012) also worked with family archives in the US: both show that the idea of the" forgotten pandemic" does not work on the family or community level. When you lose your father who is also the household's breadwinner, then you have to deal with a totally new situation (see also FANNING 2010). In Scandinavia, in Norway for instance, the difference in mortality and its consequences between the indigenous population—for instance the Sami ethnic group—and the ethnically Norwegian population was really important during the influenza pandemic. In many countries, social inequalities worsened despite the narrative of influenza as a "democratic disease" that long prevailed because statisticians couldn't really demonstrate, as they did in the 19th century for tuberculosis, that influenza was a social disease. But in 1918–1920, if everyone was susceptible to the virus because we know retrospectively that it was a "new" virus, not everyone was equally exposed. We have the same with Covid-19: it depends on your occupation, where you live, your access to care, etc. Who can work from home and follow the public health recommendations and who cannot? The social world of health care comes back: social distancing measures are interesting phenomena because they are based on science, but totally ignore the everyday life of large parts of the population. What they dismiss is the social inequalities in health among communities, which is reflected in your body, your occupation, your age, and your access to healthcare.

Something striking to me when working on the French case is that, in 1918-1919, the influenza pandemic was only one episode embedded in many different events. People had so many other issues to deal with: the last military offensives, the reconstruction of the country ... the pandemic was not the main headline. All the northern part of France was totally ravaged by the war and you had 1.4 million people who died during the Great War: there was a great shadow of death and mourning hiding the pandemic. It does not mean that the pandemic was forgotten: 50 years later, you can listen to the testimony in the recording of the radio broadcast of ROBERT DEBRÉ (1973), one of the leading medical practitioners in the country after 1945; he recounts how vivid and awful his memory is of the flu when he was a young military doctor in Tours in 1918.

Janina Kehr & Ehler Voss Current media play an incredibly important role in the Corona pandemic. And we can hardly grasp how they influence experience and action on so many levels. What role did the media play in 1918? Are there differences from and/or similarities to today? The media landscape back then is probably difficult to compare with today.

Frédéric Vagneron During the spring of 1918, there is a massive German offensive on the Western front, and the French censorship controls most of the news circulating in the public since 1915. As a consequence, the name Spanish flu, which circulated in the news at the end of the spring, reflected this desire not to demoralize public opinion during the war, by designating an epidemic event abroad. Yet, in the archive, a massive but mild influenza epidemic is mentioned in the troops in April, May, and June 1918. During the summer of 1918, some information about the epidemic in France is emerging. The main narrative

is "We do have the flu in France, it is a European epidemic, but don't worry it is worse in Germany." And the telegraphic information network also informs the population of the pandemic elsewhere in the world. A pandemic is a global event only if you know that societies are affected in many areas of the world: the Spanish flu, like the Russian flu pandemic in 1889-1890, was broadcasted by the new worldwide telegraphic network built at the end of the 19th century. From September on, there is an avalanche of information in the news. In France, censorship is less strict because the authorities feel that from August on, they are going to win the war and the magnitude of the epidemic becomes difficult to hide. The medical controversies about the epidemic and the nature of the disease, the diversity of and often contradictory medical advice make the epidemic exist in public opinion. In that sense, all the scientific controversies that we have been facing since 2020 are something not really new.

But, when you study one epidemic, you need to keep in mind the risk of singling out this specific event and cutting its many ties to previous events. In my PhD, I worked on the Spanish flu. But it was inseparable from the memory of the previous pandemic, the Russian flu of 1889-1890. The memory of the Russian flu was pretty much still there and framed many discussions in 1918 in the press, but also in the memory of individuals. For instance, the first doctors in France who identified the flu on a clinical level, very early in April-May 1918, didn't have any knowledge of the virus at the time in 1918; the virus research starts in the '30s; so the first understanding that they were possibly facing an influenza pandemic in 1918 came from older physicians who had dealt with the Russian flu, 28 years before. During the Russian flu, there were many big controversies in the medical community about the etiology of the epidemic disease. These older doctors were very vigilant in 1918: there was no conclusive bacteriological proof at hand, but the complex clinical picture of the disease during the spring of 1918 looked like what they faced in December 1889. At the time, they had dismissed the severity of some cases of influenza and the consequences of such a "popular", even if not very lethal disease.

What I want to highlight is that you have to be careful, because you want to single out what is going on now, just like when you are working on the Spanish flu you could think all the story is in the archives of 1918–1919. But the experience of the people is also a historical one; they do have a memory of their own, and it frames the event. Of course, if you bring this layer of historical experience of individuals, even when all the world is somehow struck by a similar disease, then it has a lot more complexity from one country to the other.

Janina Kehr & Ehler Voss Back in 1918, it was quite difficult for doctors to get a clear clinical picture of the disease and thus to write death certificates. The so-called bacteriological revolution was still ongoing, but viruses as such were unknown. How were the natural causes of the disease established? How did a clinical picture of the disease emerge? Which actors participated in the establishment of disease classification and based on what knowledge? Also, was there a discussion of mild vs. severe forms of disease, like we can see today? And, given that viruses were not discovered yet, what *was* the Spanish flu in 1918 and as what does it count today? What do you think about the question of retrospective diagnosis?

Frédéric Vagneron Here you need to make a detour through the social history of disease. To quote Andrew Cunningham (2002), what is the identity of the disease at the beginning of the 20th century after the so-called bacteriological revolution? Influenza is an interesting case because it was too complex to be "reduced" by the laboratory knowledge of the new germ theory ("one germ = one disease"): you have many controversies between bacteriologists, epidemiologists, and clinicians in the 1890s after the Russian flu, because they disagree about the role of the potential causative agent, the environment, or the individual terrain. With the laboratory revolution, medicine is moving to a more etiological perspective and the pursuit of the invisible causes of disease. Influenza fueled debates among the different medical disciplines. The clinicians referred to historical accounts and to the specific clinical picture of influenza, especially with the sudden fever at the onset of the sickness in comparison with mild winter colds. The bacteriologists tried to single out one causative agent. The

Pfeiffer bacillus was once thought to be the influenza microbe: only later did scientists show that this microbe was in fact what we call now *haemophiles influenzae*. It is a common bacterium in the complication of influenza. The statisticians were really important, too. Their question was simple: how do you count a case of influenza? It is a similar debate we had with Covid-19, and a way to assess the burden of the disease is to count excess mortality. The statistician raises the issue of the complications related to the influenza infection. This debate has practical consequences. In the medical community in France in 1918, there was a wide consensus that influenza is not so important as a cause of death: what actually kills you is pneumonia, bronchopneumonia, etc.

All these debates came back during the Spanish flu pandemic. Was it a mild or severe disease? The debate raged about the etiology of the disease in the medical profession. Was it severe in most cases? Was the worsening situation during the autumn of 1918 related to an increase in the unknown microbe's virulence, or to the propagation of opportunistic diseases, or to environmental factors, or to the deprivation of the population during the war? Should the medical and sanitary institutions focus on prophylaxis against influenza or on the prevention of opportunistic diseases in hospital following a primary infection? The controversies in the medical communities were one of the main forms in which the pandemic drew attention in the news. One very specific signature of the disease in 1918 was the huge death toll among the young adult population. Most of the severe cases afflicted those between 18 and 60 years old, according to the statistics. This fact was highlighted at the time and it is, of course, an epidemiological feature very different from the situation with Covid-19 and its affinity with the elderly and people with comorbidities.

Janina Kehr & Ehler Voss Numbers, thresholds, and models largely determine current national and international public health strategies to manage the Corona pandemic. Where does this "trust in numbers", to cite Theodore Porter's work (1995), come from? Was this already established in 1918? What, in your point of view, has since changed?

Frédéric Vagneron The role of statistics is really important in the public sphere from the 19th century on. A basic question with these numbers circulating everywhere is: what are you counting and what for?

We need to go back to what "counting" mortality means practically. This person is dead from Covid, this one is not, this one is likely to have died. If you count Covid-19's mortality or the Spanish flu's mortality, you are supposed to count what is written on the death certificate (CUNNINGHAM 2002). But what you write on the death certificate depends on where you are. There are huge discrepancies in the world in 1918–1919. Why do you have the 50 to 100 million gap in the mortality of 1918? Because we have no idea about what happened in countries with no or very weak systems of death certificates and mortality registration. This impressive estimate of more than 50 million deaths is a construction of retrospective surveys made in the 20th century. During the 1918–1919 pandemic, the death toll was not precisely updated every day, as has been calculated since January 2020. But in 1918 as in 2022, it is striking how difficult it is to count the dead: it is an administrative, scientific, and political operation that cruelly shows social and political inequalities on a global scale.

With a new disease such as Covid, how the death is attributed to this new disease on the certificate is obviously crucial. What is needed is some infrastructure and some kind of agreement among the people who are counting. Historically, the WHO has been one of the main institutions trying to standardize this. In February 2020, a WHO committee working on the classification of disease tried to synthesize what the identity of the disease was, to go back to Cunningham, so that medical doctors and public health officers could write Covid-19 in Lusaka and St. Petersburg with the same clinical and pathological features in mind. But this official classification does not solve everything when you have comorbidities, especially if the most susceptible people are the elderly. It's becoming really complex. If countries are not collecting the mortality data in the same way, what are you going to compare? The numbers that are circulating in France are pretty accurate, thanks to the work of institutions such as the Institut national de la statistique et des études

économiques (INSEE) and the Institut national d'études démographiques (INED), which have great experience in this matter. At the beginning, they even may have attributed too many deaths to Covid-19. Which is very different in Russia, for instance, where the authorities acknowledged at the beginning of 2021 that up to one third of Covid-19 mortality was not included in the official statistics (GUILMOTO 2022; TAYLOR 2022).

The level of "trust in numbers", of course, is totally different from one country to the other. And here I'm only discussing that through the lens of the reliability of the system. More general questions arise about your trust in your government and how governments behaved during previous crises. Some countries in the world are less keen to publish their mortality figures. So, in the end: what do you compare when you use national statistics? What is the political value of benchmarking countries based on statistics coming from infrastructure that do not apply the same methods?

Janina Kehr & Ehler Voss Currently, there is often quite vague talk of deaths "by and with" Corona …

Frédéric Vagneron Managing mortality as a means to monitor the population became a political matter in the 19th century. Mortality is becoming a public tool, while the way you die, the death, is increasingly becoming a private matter in the 20th century; that's the work of Philippe Aries. This double movement is a general feature in Western countries and is related to the growing number of people dying in hospitals in the 19th century. But a crisis may develop when there is a breakdown in managing dead bodies. Then collective death can turn into a public problem again, even if the mortality is not so great, when what had become a private ritual is not handled by the authorities on either a local or a national level. That's what happened, for instance, during the Big Heat in Chicago in the '90s or in Paris in 2003 during the "Canicule crisis" (KLINENBERG 2002; KELLER 2015).

Janina Kehr & Ehler Voss In the "Corona crisis", there have been various and changing images and criteria used to justify the necessity to take non-medical protective interventions, such as keeping distance, hygiene, and wearing masks.

In the beginning, this included the goal of "flattening the curve" with corresponding graphics, then (at least in Germany) the reproduction rate became a decisive criterion, and today it is the seven-day incidence rate, and new mutations emerge as a new rationale for maintaining the measures. With which arguments and by what means were which public health measures propagated and enforced by governmental and medical institutions during the time of the Spanish flu, and were they always the same or did they change as well?

Frédéric Vagneron In 1918, because of the blurry picture of the disease, the measures that were recommended were environmental. They didn't talk about "social distancing", but people tried to avoid public meetings, they closed theaters, etc. You were ordered to clean the ground and open the windows to have some fresh air. But at the same time, because of the approaching end of the war, soldiers would come back to their homes for a week away from the battlefield to rest. Fearing social unrest, the military decided that during the influenza pandemic they could not stop these social rights because they feared that the troops might mutiny. So, the official sanitary measures were close to what we call now social distancing. But more pragmatically, in October 1918, officials allowed some big gatherings celebrating the victory in the war. The authorities not only managed the epidemic, but also public opinion: preventing people from gathering, yes, but not if it would interfere with the celebration of the nation's victory in the war, which would risk fueling the troops' unease.

The "flattening the curve" metaphor is really related to statistical knowledge and the use of mathematical models. At the time, mathematical "modelization" of epidemics was in its infancy. Sir Ronald Ross proposed the first example of modelization a couple of years before in relation to the transmission of malaria. It became more central a little bit later with the work of KERMACK & MCKENDRICK (1927) on the now-famous R0 (basic reproduction number). Flattening the curve aims to limit the spread and the number of deaths, but it also limits the tension in hospital capacity measured by the number of beds. This question of the availability of beds was im-

portant in 1918, too. But not with a hospital infrastructure such as what we have today in the wealthiest countries, built after World War 2 and the "therapeutic revolution". Should people go to the hospital or not? It was really controversial in 1918. Some doctors said, "Yes," to care for patients with complications, for instance. Others would disagree for fear that hospitals would be overwhelmed and the risk to see the hospital transformed into a source or breeding ground of the epidemic.

Janina Kehr & Ehler Voss In the course of the current protests against the measures to contain SARS-CoV-2, we have learned that there was also a movement against wearing masks in 1918, especially in San Francisco. How common were these protests in other parts of the world, and what arguments were used to explain the rejection? Was there criticism of other measures beyond wearing masks, and if so, what were the arguments? And were there debates in different publics, as there are today, about assessing the harmfulness of the disease?

Frédéric Vagneron The first historian who mentioned the story of the anti-mask league, in my opinion, is again ALFRED CROSBY. He was a really fine historian, and this episode really belongs to the American experience with the flu and the American narrative. To my knowledge, it happened only in California and only for a short time. This shows the degree to which the memory of the Spanish flu in 2021 is recalled as an American experience. The anti-mask league was really an exception in the world for a simple reason: not so many people wore masks, almost none. In Lausanne, Switzerland, you had a public campaign for people to wear masks; in France, it was already a debate among bacteriologists and hygienists. Some of them were really trying to provide scientific evidence of the preventive role of the mask. They experimented with patients coughing and a series of petri dishes at one meter, at two meters, etc. to measure how far expelled droplets would travel. These experiments were tied to the recommendation to wear masks. But recommending masks and producing them in quantity are two different things. Today you can imagine that in 1918 everyone was wearing a mask. In Europe, I don't think it was the case, and I never read it was the case in Africa or South America. Japan may well have been another exception. Public health reports on the national level in 1919 present wearing a mask as a means to avoid the disease. In 1918, protests came from workers in theaters, who wrote letters or petitions asking the mayors to help them during the closure of their workplace. In these letters, sometimes published in the press, they do not really challenge the public health rationale for the closure, but merely ask for public support.

It is not so different from today with lockdown policies. But in 1918, only small parts of the population were directly impacted by these sanitary measures. With the Covid-19 lockdown policies in many countries, this has happened on a totally different scale.

Janina Kehr & Ehler Voss As a historian who has examined the media on the 1918 epidemic, you have often been confronted with the question what we can learn from the 1918 flu. We do not wish to reiterate this question, but rather to turn it around: how and why, from your point of view, has the 1918 flu become the blueprint for Covid-19? What problems do you see in such comparisons?

Frédéric Vagneron There is indeed an important narrative in the media and among public health experts today drawing on the so-called "lessons of the past". What can we learn from the 1918 management of the pandemic? Many newspapers described in 2020 how many people used masks in 1918/1919 and the mitigation policies in different countries, in the US and elsewhere. Most of the time, these accounts focus on one object, one location, one measure and try to draw parallels with our current situation to explain what we should do and asking in what ways we are better or worse. But "lessons" about what? What kind of common experience of the flu in 1918 in France, Germany, the US and elsewhere? Forging an artificial common experience to serve as a template to establish or enforce our contemporary policies is a simplistic way to use history. It's not answers and successful tools we can learn from the past, but unsolved questions that this uneven experience raises. How do you communicate in

a time of uncertainty? How do you build confidence in a public health infrastructure when the system is drained by financial cuts or weakened by a shortage of personnel? How do you build a public health response that both shares the costs of a pandemic but also provides a flexible local response that fits the local challenge that a global pandemic poses? How do you deal with a disease that can cause a very mild sickness as well as severe cases and large numbers of fatalities? That's not "lessons of the past", but challenges from the past, from a totally different context. I don't see how we can find ready-made recipes from 1918 when nobody had "modern" scientific understanding of viruses. But I see many interesting ways to think, using some questions from the past.

To go back to your question: influenza has been an important historical precedent in the 20th century because it was a viral disease that could not be directly controlled during a large part of the 20th century. But the influenza pandemic of 1918–1919 was not a major blow to the modern narrative of scientific progress and the long-term victory over infectious diseases in Western countries. Influenza escaped the so-called "therapeutic revolution" after 1945, even if the bacterial complications of influenza could now be dealt with. But it was not possible to prevent the 1957 Asian flu or the 1968 or the 1997 Hong Kong flu from happening periodically. Influenza remained a moving target during most of the 20th century and fueled the pandemic narrative in Western countries, where the burden and the common experience of infectious diseases progressively disappeared.

The memory of the 1918 flu pandemic became more salient in the 1970s and during the HIV/AIDS pandemic: remember the new title of the second edition of ALFRED CROSBY's book when it was published again in the mid-1980s: "Epidemic and Peace", a very contextual title, became "The Forgotten Pandemic". Historians then gained the status of experts in the public health agenda when the label "emerging diseases" gained some traction after the 1989 conference in Washington, D.C. WILLIAM H. MCNEIL (1976) and other historians participated along with biomedical experts, sharing their expertise on the history of pandemic events (MORSE 1993). The same thing happened with anthropologists working during the HIV/AIDS pandemic to combat the population's irrational "resistance" to science and to foster "acceptance" of public measures … sometimes also participating in the stigmatization of the population (FASSIN 1999). The expertise of the social sciences in health dates back to this period of the early 1980s. In the 1990s, influenza and influenza pandemics became a global model of the threat that could come from anywhere in the world because of its animal origins. The influenza pandemic became the blueprint of the global threat that (wealthy) countries had to be prepared for. That also includes special features of public health influenza campaigns, such as the challenge to vaccination with its many strains. This has, of course, some echo today with the mutations and variants of Covid-19. Thus, influenza can also be a template for studying the contemporary vaccine hesitancy.

References

BRISTOW, NANCY K. 2012. *American Pandemic. The Lost Worlds of the 1918 Influenza Epidemic*. New York: Oxford University Press.

CROSBY, ALFRED W. 1976. *Epidemic and Peace, 1918*. Westport: Greenwood Press.

—— 1989 *America's Forgotten Pandemic. The Influenza of 1918*. New York: Cambridge University Press.

CUNNINGHAM, ANDREW 2002. Identifying Diseases in the Past: Cutting through the Gordian Knot. *Asclepio* 54, 13–34.

—— 1992. Transforming plague. The laboratory and the identity of infectious disease. In CUNNINGHAM, ANDREW & WILLIAMS, PERRY (eds). *The Laboratory Revolution in Medicine*. Cambridge: Cambridge University Press: 9–44.

DEBRÉ, ROBERT 1973. Interview. In LALLIER, JEAN & TOSELLO, MONIQUE (prod). *Un flžau familier: la grippe*, Radio Show Portrait de l'Univers.

FANNING, PATRICIA J. 2010. *Influenza and Inequality. One Town's Tragic Response to the Great Epidemic of 1918*. Amherst: University of Massachusetts Press.

FARGE, ARLETTE 2019. *Vies oubliées. Au coeur du XVIIIe siècle*. Paris: La Découverte.

FASSIN, DIDIER 1999. L'anthropologie entre engagement et distanciation. Essai de sociologie des recherches en sciences sociales sur le sida en Afrique. In BECKER, CHARLES; DOZON, JEAN-PIERRE; OBBO, CHRISTINE & TOURÉ, MORIBA (eds) *Vivre et penser le sida en Afrique*. Dakar, Paris: Codesira, Karthala, IRD: 41–66.

GUILMOTO, CHRISTOPHE Z. 2022. An alternative estimation of the death toll of the Covid-19 pandemic in India. *PLoS ONE* 17, 2: e0263187. https://doi.org/10.1371/journal.pone.0263187.

JOHNSON, NIALL P. A. S. & MUELLER, JUERGEN 2002. Updating the accounts. Global mortality of the 1918–1920 "Spanish" influenza pandemic, *Bulletin of the History of Medicine* 76,1: 105–115.

JONES, ESYLLT W. 2007. *Influenza 1918. Disease, Death, and Struggle in Winnipeg*. Toronto: University of Toronto Press.

KELLER, RICHARD C. 2015. *Fatal Isolation. The Devastating Paris Heat Wave of 2003*. Chicago: University of Chicago Press.

KERMACK, WILLIAM OGILVY & MCKENDRICK, ANDERSON GRAY 1927. A contribution to the mathematical theory of epidemics. *Proceedings of the Royal Society of London* A 115, 772: 700–721.

KLINENBERG, ERIC 2002. *Heat Wave. A Social Autopsy of Disaster in Chicago*. Chicago: University of Chicago Press.

LAQUEUR, THOMAS W. 2015. *The Work of the Dead. A Cultural History of Mortal Remains*. Princeton: Princeton University Press.

MCNEILL, WILLIAM H. 1976. *Plagues and Peoples*. Garden City, New York: Anchor Press, Doubleday.

MORSE, STEPHEN S. (ed) 1993. *Emerging Viruses*. Oxford: Oxford University Press.

PORTER, THEODORE M. 1995. *Trust in Numbers. The Pursuit of Objectivity in Science and Public Life*. Princeton: Princeton University Press.

ROSENBERG, CHARLES E. 1989. What is an epidemic? AIDS in historical perspective. *Daedalus* 118, 2: 1–17.

TAYLOR, LUKE 2022. Covid-19. True global death toll from pandemic is almost 15 million, says WHO. *BMJ*: 377.

VAGNERON, FRÉDÉRIC 2022. Morts et enterrés. La gestion des morts durant la grippe espagnole en France (1918–1919). In SENIK, CLAUDIA (ed) *Pandémies. Nos sociétés à l'épreuve*. Paris: La Découverte: 121–138.

JANINA KEHR | Univ.-Prof. Dr., is a professor of medical anthropology and global health in the Department of Social and Cultural Anthropology at the University of Vienna. Her work is concerned with global infectious diseases, hospital spaces and places, medicine and the economy, and, more recently, the environmental impact of technoscientific biomedicine. She focuses on the temporal hauntings, moral economies, and multiple inequalities in contemporary healthcare systems, particularly in Europe.

University of Vienna, Department of Social and Cultural Anthropology
Universitätsstraße 7, 1030 Vienna, Austria
janina.kehr@univie.ac.at

FRÉDÉRIC VAGNERON | Dr., is a historian of medicine and science and a lecturer at the University of Strasbourg, affiliated with the SAGE research laboratory. His main field of research is the history of infectious diseases from a perspective combining the social history of knowledge and epidemics. His current work focuses on the relationships between human health and animal health in the second half of the 20th century.

University of Strasbourg, Department of Science and Medicine History (DHVS)
Faculté de médecine, 4 rue Kirschleger, 67085 Strasbourg, France
fvagneron@unistra.fr

EHLER VOSS | Dr., is an anthropologist with a focus on the intersections of medical anthropology, media anthropology, political anthropology, and the anthropology of religion. With reference to Science and Technology Studies, he focuses on the intersections of scientific, religious, and medical lay and expert cultures from the perspective of pop-cultural and political practices and issues and examines the transatlantic entanglements of orthodox and heterodox knowledge cultures from the 19th century to the present.

University of Bremen, RTG Contradiction Studies
Grazer Straße 2, 28359 Bremen, Germany
ehler.voss@uni-bremen.de

Forschungspraxis, Diskriminierungsformen und Handlungsmöglichkeiten in der Pflege, Versorgung und Betreuung von trans*-Kindern und -Jugendlichen

Ein Forschungsbericht

MANUEL BOLZ & SABINE WÖHLKE

Abstract In unserem Forschungsbericht stellen wir unser empirisches Forschungsdesign, erste Ergebnisse des Verbundprojektes TRANS*KIDS und des Hamburger Teilprojektes vor. Unser Projekt hat zum Ziel, (potenzielle) Diskriminierungen und Stigmatisierungen von professionell Pflegenden und (medizinischen) Fach- und Verwaltungsangestellten in Kliniken und in Ärzt*innenpraxen im Umgang mit trans*-Kindern und -Jugendlichen herauszuarbeiten. Diese, so zeigt es unsere Auswertung, zeigen sich als Hindernis für eine wertschätzende, diversitäts- und geschlechtssensible Pflege, Betreuung und Versorgung. Der Beitrag fungiert als Werkstattbericht um die Forschungspraxis, das Material und die Methode vorzustellen, zu diskutieren und kritisch zu evaluieren.

Schlagwörter Geschlechtsidentität – Pflege – medizinische Verwaltung – Gesundheitsversorgung – Diskriminierung

Einführung. Gesundheit und Geschlechtsidentität in der Gegenwart

Der folgende Beitrag stellt ein Forschungsbericht des Verbundprojektes TRANS*KIDS und des Hamburger Teilprojektes dar, indem das empirische Forschungsdesign und erste Ergebnisse der Auswertung vorgestellt werden. Untersucht wurden bewusste und unbewusste Diskriminierungen von Pflegefachkräften sowie medizinischen Fach- und Verwaltungsangestellten im Umgang mit trans*-Kinder und -Jugendlichen.

Menschen, die in der Gegenwartsgesellschaft aufgrund einer dominant männlichen und cisheteronormativ-orientierten Ausrichtung als „anders" markiert werden, sind gefährdet, in der Gesundheitsversorgung und -förderung diskriminiert und stigmatisiert zu werden. Berufsgruppen der Gesundheitsversorgung wie Pflegende, medizinische Fach- und Verwaltungsangestellte können – durch strukturelle Hindernisse gehemmte – Kompetenzen fehlen, um mit trans*-Patient*innen sensibel umzugehen. Auch die Covid-19-Pandemie hatte Konsequenzen für unser Forschungsfeld im Gesundheitswesen, verstärkte Grenzziehungen und Ausschließungen. In medialen Diskursen werden Gesundheitsberufe mit Beginn der Pandemie im März 2020 als „systemrelevant" eingestuft und über unterschiedlichste Anerkennungsformen (monetär, sozial und ideell) entlohnt. Mitunter waren es polarisierende, emotionalisierende und moralisierende Debatten, welche die Notwendigkeiten einer wertschätzenden Pflege, Betreuung und Versorgung zementierten (vgl. MÖLLER, GÜLDENRING, WIESEMANN & ROMER 2018). In der Pandemie waren es vor allem vulnerable Gruppen (wie zum Beispiel trans*-Akteur*innen), deren Zugänge zur Gesundheitsversorgung durch spezifische Ein- und Ausschlussmechanismen geprägt waren: fehlende finanzielle Ressourcen und prekäre Lebenslagen, infrastrukturell schwach ausgebaute Wohnorte, fehlende Mobilitätsformen und Versorgungsangebote, fehlende soziale Netzwerke und Infrastrukturen, vorhandene sprachliche Barrieren und emotionale Zustände zum Beispiel Ängste oder Ungewissheiten (vgl. JENNER 2010; WEISS 2019; ROWE, CHYE & O'KEEFE 2019).[1]

Vor diesem Hintergrund arbeiten wir im Projekt zum einen Herausforderungen, Potenziale und Grenzen des Forschens in medizinischen Forschungsfeldern um trans*-Identität unter Pandemiebedingungen heraus, zum anderen kartieren wir die Netzwerke und Akteur*innenkonstellationen, Gesundheitsinstitutionen und -infrastrukturen, biomedizinische Wissensregime und Biopolitiken, die in der Pflege, der Behandlung und Versorgung von trans*-Kindern und -Jugendlichen relevant sind. Dabei konzentrieren wir uns auf spezifische Lebenswirklichkeiten, Erfahrungswelten und Wissensbestände von im Gesundheitswesen Tätigen. Wir hinterfragen die normativen Ordnungsprinzipien, die dem Gesundheitssystem und ihren Vorstellungen von physischer und psychischer Gesundheit und Krankheit zu Grunde liegen. Dies tun wir auch, um die Argumentationsgrundlagen nachzuzeichnen und kritisch einzuordnen, die politische Prozesse um trans* prägen und nach wie vor handlungsleitend sind: Psycho(patho)logisierungen und Medikalisierungsprozesse.[2]

Die Covid-19-Pandemie hat demnach auch auf transidente Menschen erhebliche Auswirkungen zur Folge, da sich die Gefahr der Mehrfachdiskriminierungen und Stigmatisierung verstärkt hat (vgl. EUROPEAN UNION AGENCY FOR FUNDAMENTAL RIGHTS 2014: 42ff; GÜLDENRING 2015; KRELL & OLDEMEIER 2016). Die Betroffenenvertretungen nennen zum Beispiel die Verstärkung von psychosozialen Auswirkungen der pandemischen Zustände auf trans*-Personen, vor allem auf trans*-Kinder und -Jugendliche, so beispielsweise veränderte Familienbeziehungen, häusliche Gewaltformen (zu sexualisierter Gewalt vgl. DU MONT, KOSA, SOLOMON & MACDONALD 2019; LSVD 2022), Einreiseverbote und fehlende Kontaktmöglichkeiten, die zu Gefühlen der Einsamkeit und Situationen der Isolation führen konnten. Aber auch im medizinischen Bereich bzw. im Gesundheitsbereich betreffen die Auswirkungen der Pandemie Geschlechtsidentitäten, Formen der Körperarbeit, verzögerte oder abgesagte Unterstützungsmaßnahmen für Transitionsprozesse und fehlende Vernetzungsmöglichkeiten, weil die Anlaufstellen von Selbsthilfegruppen und Beratungsstellen aufgrund von Abstandsregelungen und Ansteckungsgefahren geschlossen und Termine bei Psychotherapeut*innen ausgesetzt wurden (vgl. SZÜCS, KÖHLER, HOLTHAUS, GÜLDENRING, BALK, MOT-

MANS & NIEDER 2021; DEUTSCHER BUNDESTAG 2022).

Es wird deutlich: Die Pandemie führte wie ein Brennglas vor Augen, wie prekär und brüchig die pflegerische Versorgung, Begleitung und Betreuung von hilfsbedürftigen Menschen in unserem Gesundheitssystem ist. Trans*-Kinder und -Jugendliche stellen hier eine vulnerable Gruppe dar, da sie mit ihren Bedürfnissen nicht in der medizinischen Rangordnung eines Krisennotfallmanagements als besonders akut eingestuft werden. Nichtsdestotrotz sollten trans*-Personen keinesfalls als homogene Gruppe oder als rein passiv verstanden werden. Im Gegenteil, sie entwickelten gerade in Krisenzuständen wie der Pandemie kreative, teilweise auch subversive Handlungsstrategien der Selbstsorge und Resilienz. Sie bildeten u. a. regionale Gesundheitsnetzwerke. Eine medizinanthropologische Analyse setzt in diesem Spannungs- und Konfliktfeld an und legt Fremd- und Selbstbilder von Patient*innen und von spezifischen Arbeitskulturen offen (vgl. CARABEZ, PELLEGRINI, MANKOVITZ, ELIASON & DARIOTIS 2015).

Die Hürden für trans*-Patient*innen, medizinische Versorgungs- und Vorsorgepraktiken wahrzunehmen oder gar Zugänge zu Wissensressourcen zu erhalten, verstärkten sich und beeinflussten auch unsere Forschung. Des Weiteren prägte das Pandemiegeschehen nicht nur die Rekrutierung und Materialerhebung, sondern darüber hinaus auch die Dynamiken und Eigenlogiken der Forschungsfelder im Gesundheitssystem, vor allem durch die entstandenen Mehrfachbelastungen. Denn durch die Pandemie verschärften sich die ohnehin schon desolaten Arbeitsbedingungen teilweise erheblich. Dies resultierte in einer mangelhaften Versorgung, Betreuung und Pflege der Patient*innen.

Die Psychologie und die Sozialwissenschaften haben den Ansatz des *minority stress* (zu Deutsch: *Minderheitenstress*) als ein machtvolles Deutungsmuster herausgearbeitet. Dies wurde durch gendertheoretische Perspektiven ergänzt (vgl. ROOD, REISNER, SURACE, PUCKETT, MARONEY & PANTALONE 2016; HUNTER, BUTLER & COOPER 2021; TOOMEY 2021). Damit werden ineinandergeflochtene Stresssituationen benannt, die vor allem vulnerable Gruppen wie trans*-Kinder und -Jugendliche im Alltag erfahren bzw. mit denen sie aufgrund von Stigmatisierungen, Diskriminierungen und Positionierungen im sozialen Feld unfreiwillig konfrontiert sind. Dazu gehören auch als negativ empfundene Erfahrungen im Gesundheitssystem und in Ärzt*innenpraxen, gerade, wenn sie diese ohne Sorgeberechtigte passieren. Dies kann dazu führen, dass trans*-Kinder und -Jugendliche weitere ärztliche Termine nicht alleine wahrnehmen möchten. Des Weiteren prägen solche negativen Erfahrungen im Gesundheitswesen das Bild vom Gesundheitssystem insgesamt nachhaltig. Hier schließen Fragen danach an, welchen Stellenwert die Transidentität annimmt, wenn transunspezifische Behandlungen durchgeführt werden sollen und wie die Wahrnehmung solcher Gesundheitsmaßnahmen emotional aufgeladen oder gar abgelehnt werden.

Es lässt sich also resümieren, dass es nicht nur psychologische, sondern vor allem soziale Gefüge sind, die solche Stresssituationen hervorbringen und die Zerrbilder über Behandlungen und Diagnose prägen. Ferner können auch Pflegefachkräfte und medizinische Fach- und Verwaltungsangestellte emotionale, moralische, psychische und physische Stresssituationen erleiden (vgl. WÖHLKE & WIESEMANN 2016).

Die leitfadengestützten, semi-strukturierten Interviews konzentrierten sich im Rahmen des Projektes auf (potentielle) Diskriminierungen, Herabsetzungen und Herabwürdigungen von trans*-Patient*innen im Arbeitsalltag, obwohl sicherlich auch andere Formen der Kommunikation und Interaktion im Gesundheitswesen eine Rolle spielen können. Die Interviews fungieren als spezifische Medien, über das eigene biografische Arbeits- und Erfahrungswissen zu sprechen, es retrospektiv zu ordnen und zu strukturieren (vgl. STUCKEY 2013; HOPF 2019). Die Erzählungen über arbeitsspezifisches Erfahrungswissen liegen uns nicht in „Reinform" vor, sondern sind bereits gefiltert, durch Auslassungen und Akzentuierungen gekennzeichnet. Uns geht es daher nicht darum, die Äußerungen auf ihren Wahrheitsgehalt zu prüfen, sie also als „richtig" oder „falsch" einzuordnen oder zu bewerten. Vielmehr wollen wir aufzeigen, was als erzähl- und erinnerungswürdig gedeutet wird und wie Darstellungsweisen von Wissen über Diskriminierung, Stigmatisierung und

Herausforderungen im Arbeitsalltag als sinnhaft gestaltet werden: Sie prägen Argumentations- und Erzählleitlinien und eigene Berufsverständnisse. Die Anerkennung des situierten und prozessualen Wissens bedeutet deshalb, objektive Wissenschaftsverständnisse in den Lebens- und Gesundheitswissenschaften aufzubrechen (für eine feministische Epistemologie siehe HARAWAY 1995). Denn das akademische Wissen ist immer auch abhängig von den Prozessen, Instrumenten und Wertvorstellungen ihrer Hervorbringung. Das Projekt möchte deshalb dafür sensibilisieren, dass medizinische Wissenskulturen nicht neutral sind und akteur*innenzentrierte Erfahrungen, Wahrnehmungen, Körper- und Geschlechtsverständnisse in alltäglichen Arbeitsroutinen und in der Wissensvermittlung berücksichtigt werden sollten. Des Weiteren weisen wir auf die Verstärkung von Diskriminierungsmechanismen, dichotome Menschenbilder im Gesundheitssystem und auf die Gleichzeitigkeit von Geschlechterentwürfen in Arbeitspraktiken und -routinen hin.

In diesem Bericht reflektieren wir unsere Forschungspraxis des Hamburger Teilprojektes des Verbundprojektes TRANS*KIDS während der Covid-19-Pandemie und arbeiten erste Diskriminierungs- und Stigmatisierungsdimensionen heraus.[3] Nachdem die Hintergründe des Teilprojektes verdeutlicht wurden, erläutern wir im nächsten Schritt das Forschungsdesign. Die empirische Phase unseres Teilprojektes fand ausschließlich unter den Bedingungen und Veränderungen von Covid-19 statt, so dass unmittelbare Einblicke in pflegerische und verwaltungstechnische Arbeitsalltage und -kulturen durch teilnehmende Beobachtungen nicht möglich waren. Zentral erscheint uns hier die Frage, wie in Zeiten von Abstandsregelungen, Ansteckungsrisiken und Ausgangsbeschränkungen qualitativ-empirische Forschung in medizinischen Forschungsfeldern durchgeführt werden kann, besonders, wenn sich Arbeitsalltage durch die Pandemie erheblich verändert haben. Abschließend stellen wir erste Ergebnisse unserer Analyse des empirischen Materials vor und zeigen die Verwobenheiten zwischen der individuellen, institutionellen und strukturellen Ebene im Gesundheitswesen (vgl. TEZCAN-GÜNTEKIN 2020). Hier schließt auch die Frage an, welche Diskriminirungen und Herausforderungen trans*- und/oder altersspezifisch sind und welche nicht (vgl. MEDINA, MAHOWALD, SANTOS & GURBERG 2021; HÄDICKE & WIESEMANN 2021). Geschlechtsidentität/trans*im Gesundheitswesen ist ein sehr umkämpftes Feld, vor allem was medizinische Deutungshoheiten angeht. Durch die Literaturdichte und die internationalen Verweise auf sozial- und gesundheitswissenschaftliche Studien möchten wir die Aufmerksamkeit auf die Leerstellen und blinden Flecken innerhalb der deutschsprachigen Forschungslandschaft lenken. In der Entwicklung von Maßnahmen zum Abbau von Mehrfachdiskriminierung dürfen die internationalen Vergleiche nicht unberücksichtigt bleiben. Auch die trans*-Communities selbst haben Wissen und Strategien produziert, die es im Sinne von partizipativer Gesundheitsforschung zu integrieren gilt. Das Spannungsfeld der Wissensaufbereitung als Interventionsform erstreckt sich demnach zwischen Wissenschaft, Politik und Aktivismus.

Das Forschungsdesign des Projekts TRANS*KIDS

Der vom Bundesministerium für Gesundheit (BMG) geförderte Forschungsverbund *TRANS*-KIDS* ist ein Projekt zur Förderung eines nichtdiskriminierenden Umgangs mit jungen trans*-Kindern und -Jugendlichen durch patient*innenorientierte Schulungs-, Lehr- und Weiterbildungsmaßnahmen im Gesundheitswesen.[4] Das heißt, das generierte Wissen wird aufbereitet, zitierbar gemacht und in didaktische, visuell-gestützte Vermittlungskonzepte und Repräsentationsformen übersetzt (vgl. KNECHT 2013; GAJEK 2014). Fallbeispiele und Vignetten werden darüber hinaus mit Ansätzen des *Blended Learning* und des Forschenden Lernen verknüpft, um einzelne Arbeitswelten zu explizieren (vgl. DÍAZ, MARUCA, GONZALEZ, STOCKMANN, HOYT & BLACKWELL 2017; MCCAVE, APTAKER, HARTMANN & ZUCCONI 2019).

Das Verbundprojekt ist dreigeteilt: Das Teilprojekt an der Westfälischen Wilhelms-Universität Münster erhebt sowohl qualitative als auch quantitative Daten. Mithilfe von leitfadengestützten Interviews und Fragebögen wurden trans*-Kinder, -Jugendliche und deren Sorgeberechtigten befragt sowie Fokusgruppen durch-

geführt, um die Ergebnisse zu evaluieren und zu diskutieren (vgl. BROKMEIER, MUCHA, ROMER & FÖCKER 2022; MUCHA, BROKMEIER, RAREY, ROMER & FÖCKER 2022; MUCHA, BROKMEIER, RAREY, ROMER & FÖCKER O. A.). Das Teilprojekt am Institut für Ethik und Geschichte der Medizin der Georg-August-Universität Göttingen hat mittels leitfadengestützter Interviews medizinische Fachexpert*innen befragt (zum Beispiel Kinderärzt*innen, Psycholog*innen, Endokrinolog*innen etc.) (vgl. WIESEMANN 2020). Das hier im Fokus des Beitrages stehende Teilprojekt der Hochschule für Angewandte Wissenschaften in Hamburg (HAW), das während der Covid-19-Pandemie im Herbst 2021 startete, hat die Gruppe der professionell Pflegenden sowie den Bereich des (medizinischen) Verwaltungspersonals, also zum Beispiel *Office Nurses*, medizinische Fachangestellte und Arzthelfer*innen im Fokus. Diese Berufsgruppen führen in der alltäglichen Pflege, Betreuung und Versorgung vermehrt Interaktions- und Kommunikationsformen mit trans*-Kindern und -Jugendlichen durch, weniger im Sinne einer Diagnosestellung, sondern in Form einer Beziehungsgestaltung (vgl. ROSA, CARVALHO, PEREIRA, ROCHA, NEVES, ROSA 2019 & THUMM 2022). Aufgrund der teilweise sehr körpernahen Arbeitserfahrungen besitzen diese Arbeitskulturen spezifisches Expert*innen- und Erfahrungswissen, das sich in Arbeitsroutinen manifestiert, gleichzeitig jedoch auf Situationen verweist, welche diskriminierend wirken können (vgl. SCHNEIDER & WÖHLKE 2022; SCHORRLEPP 2022). Das Teilprojekt nutzt einen empirisch-ethischen und medizinanthropologischen Ansatz, um sich diesen Ambivalenzen anzunähern (vgl. VAN DER DONK, VAN LANEN & WRIGHT 2014; siehe auch ZUNNER 2012; WÖHLKE & SCHICKTANZ 2019). Es knüpft damit auch an philosophisch-reflexive, medizinische, psychologische und rechtswissenschaftliche Studien an (vgl. AMELUNG 2019 und die Beiträge in APPENROTH & VARELA 2019).

Eine transsensible Pflege von Kindern und Jugendlichen, so unser Ausgangspunkt, beinhaltet eine Reflexion über internalisierte und externalisierte Normen, medizinische und psychologische Wissensbestände sowie die kritische Einordnung von gesellschaftlichen Regelsystemen. Doch wie wirkt sich eine (Un-)Ordnung des bisherigen Regelwerkes auf den kompetenten Umgang geschlechts- und diversitätssensibler Pflege aus, die in Krisenzeiten wie die Covid-19-Pandemie besonders eingefordert ist (vgl. KEEPNEWS 2011; KELLETT & FITTON 2017; SHERMAN, McDOWELL, CLARK, BALTHAZAR, KLEPPER & BOWER 2021)? Wir fragen demnach nach den (un)sichtbaren Werteverständnissen, die als Hindernis einer wertschätzenden Pflege im Sinne des Pflegekodex der *International Council of Nurses* (ICN) präsent sind, an dem sich institutionelle Setzungen und Rahmungen orientieren und die zu stigmatisierendem, diskriminierendem und herausforderndem Situationen führen können (vgl. AMERICAN NURSES ASSOCIATION (ANA) 2018).[5] SABINE WÖHLKE und ERIK SCHNEIDER (2022) verweisen in ihrem Beitrag auf die „Charta der Rechte hilfe- und pflegebedürftiger Menschen" von 2020, dass die Pflegefach und -weiterbildung die Würde und die Einzigartigkeit des Menschen in ihre theoretisch-konzeptionelle Grundsätze integriert hat. In der Praxis ist dies aber noch nicht vollständig umgesetzt, gerade wenn es um die Akzeptanz von Geschlechtsidentitäten geht. Sie unterscheiden auf der theoretischen Ebene vier Dimensionen von einem transsensiblen Pflegehandeln: regelgeleitetes, situativ-beurteilendes Handeln, reflektierendes und aktivethisches Handeln. Des Weiteren monieren sie die Lücke zwischen alltagspraktischem Handeln auf Stationen in Kliniken oder in Ärzt*innenpraxen und ihrem Arbeitsethos. Sie sind häufig nicht deckungsgleich und bedingen Abwägungs- und Aushandlungsprozesse über Umgangsweisen.

Nicht nur die Pandemiesituation, auch der Blick auf bereits bestehendes Lehr- und Praxisliteratur für die Pflegeberufe und medizinische Fach- und Verwaltungsangestellte zeigt Lücken und fehlende Wissensressourcen auf (vgl. MERRYFEATHER & BRUCE 2014): Diversität, der Pluralismus an Lebenswelten, Geschlechterentwürfen und Identitätsvorstellungen werden überwiegend mit den Zugehörigkeiten und Zuschreibungskategorien Ethnizität und Religion verbunden. Aufbereitetes Praxis- und Erfahrungswissen zu Geschlechtsidentität in Pflege- und medizinischen Verwaltungskontexten fehlt meistens oder wurde bisher nur punktuell ausgearbeitet (vgl. ALEGRIA 2011; BEAGEN & GOLDBERG 2012; CICERO & PERRY 2015; AMERICAN ACADEMY OF PEDIATRICS 2018). Auch in den Ausbildungsplänen und Curricula stellt das Thema Geschlechtsidentität wie zum Beispiel trans* nach wie vor ein Desiderat dar (vgl. FIDELINDO & BERNSTEIN 2012; FIDELINDO, BROWN, JONES 2013; McDOWELL & BOWER 2016; VOSS 2021; BÖHM & VOSS 2022 a/b). Veränderungen in den Wissensstrukturen, Vermittlungsformen und -strategien lassen sich erst in den letzten Jahren erkennen. Es lässt sich daher festhalten, dass die Wissensaufbereitung personen- und ortsabhängig und nicht systematisch oder gar nachhaltig in Bildungsinstitutionen erfolgt (vgl. NAKOMM 2022). Ferner bleibt fraglich, welche Konzepte von Transidentität und Transkulturalität in der Benennung, in der Beschreibung und im Verständnis der geschlechtsspezifischen Erfahrungswerte und Identitätskonstruktionen verwendet werden, wie trans* zu bestehenden Geschlechtsbinaritäten und zu *non-binary/agender* in Beziehung gesetzt und Geschlechtsidentität und sexuelle/romantische Orientierung fälschlicherweise synonym verwendet werden (für eine kulturanthropologische Einordnung vgl. HESS 1999). Vor allem Letzteres wird in antigenderistischen und populistischen Argumentationen aufgegriffen, um Abwehrhaltungen, Grenzziehungen und Distanzierungen zu erzeugen und Akteur*innen politisch zu mobilisieren (zum Einstieg siehe NÄSER-LATHER 2019).

Forschen unter Covid-19. Wechselwirkungen, Konflikte, Spannungsfelder

Um die Perspektive von Pflegefachkräften und medizinischen Fach- und Verwaltungsangestellten auf den Umgang mit trans*-Kindern und -Jugendlichen in Ärzt*innenpraxen, auf Stationen und in Klinikkontexten zu explorieren, nutzen wir ein qualitatives, sozialempirisches Forschungsdesign. In den Jahren 2021 und 2022 führten wir fünfzehn semistrukturierte Interviews mittels Videotelefonie (Zoom) mit einer durchschnittlichen Dauer zwischen 45 und 90 Minuten durch. Die Gespräche geben Rückschlüsse über spezifische Erfahrungen innerhalb der Arbeitskulturen und ihren Umgang mit minderjährigen trans*-Patient*innen.

Als unser Teilprojekt im September 2021 startete, arbeiteten die anderen beiden Teilprojekte bereits seit mehr als zwei Jahren. Das vorhandene Netzwerk an Kooperationspartner*innen wie beispielsweise die trans*-Communities half uns beim Feldeinstieg. Zu reflektieren gilt, dass die unterschiedlichen Akteur*innen aus Wissenschaft, Aktivismus, Bildungspolitik und Vermittlungsarbeit, deren Rollen teilweise verschwimmen, verschiedene Meinungen, Haltungen und Interessen vertreten, die sich wiederum auf Prioritäten, Ressourcenverteilung und Schwerpunktsetzungen auswirken. So werden trans*-Kindern und -Jugendlichen verschiedene Dimensionen von Verletzlichkeit/-barkeit und Selbstbestimmung zugeschrieben, die teilweise auch gegeneinander abgewogen werden. Wir identifizierten in unserem Forschungsfeld Rollenüberlagerungen: aktivistische Wissenschaftler*innen und forschende Aktivist*innen aus den Bereichen der sozialen, sexualwissenschaftlichen bzw. -pädagogischen und queer-feministischen Arbeit. Die von uns untersuchten Berufsgruppen wurden in den sozialstaatlichen Unterstützungsmaßnahmen zum Abbau von Diskriminierungen und Stigmatisierungen von trans*-Personen bisher vernachlässigt. Pflegende, Betreuende und Versorgende besitzen einen großen berufsbiographischen Wissensfundus über mögliche Risiken und Gefahren, gerade auch, weil sie tagtäglich in einer (körpernahen) Kommunikation und Interaktion mit trans*-Patient*innen stehen. Außerdem erfahren wir etwas über Momente der Überforderung und der Irritation.

Unseren Interviewaufruf streuten wir über projektinterne Netzwerke. Vorausgegangen war die Teilnahme an Netzwerktreffen und Workshops mit Kooperationspartner*innen der trans*-Community-Vertretungen sowie an digital durchgeführten regionalen Gesundheitsnetzwerktreffen, in denen wir unser Forschungsprojekt vorstellen durften. Gemeinsam mit den trans*-Communities entwickelten und evaluierten wir den Interviewleitfaden. Durch erste Pretest-Interviews (Pilotierung) mit Pflegenden erhielten wir Rückmeldungen zu den Interviewfragen und einen ersten Eindruck über die Verwobenheit individueller Betreuungsverständnisse, stationärer Arbeitsroutinen, struktureller Hindernisse und institutioneller Setzungen (Klinikrichtlinien, Rechtsprechungen oder Krankenkassen).

Die Akteur*innen meldeten sich auf den Interviewaufruf, weil sie in ihren alltäglichen Arbeitssituationen Kontakt mit trans*-Kindern und -Jugendlichen haben und diese Erfahrung teilen wollten. Doch welche Hintergründe haben unsere Interviewpartner*innen? Das Sample des Teilprojektes besteht aus insgesamt 15 Interviews, sechs Interviews mit Pflegefachkräften einer Station für Innere Medizin, aus der Kinder- und Jugendpsychiatrie, Psychotherapie und Psychosomatik, aus der Kinderpoliklinik bzw. der Kindernotaufnahme sowie aus dem Bereich von transspezifischen Sprechstunden. Des Weiteren konnten fünf Interviews mit medizinischen Fachangestellten aus einer (kinder)endokrinologischen Praxis, der Kinder- und Jugendpsychiatrie, Psychotherapie und Psychosomatik sowie der Kardiologie geführt werden. Hinzu kommen vier Gespräche mit Akteur*innen aus der Verwaltung von einer kinder-, jugendpsychiatrischen und klinischen Praxis, aus der Logopädie sowie der Kunsttherapie. Die Akteur*innen unterscheiden sich vom Alter (von Anfang zwanzig bis über sechzig Jahre), der Berufserfahrung (von unter fünf bis über dreißig Jahre), dem Standort (in ganz Deutschland verteilt, großstädtische und ländliche Regionen) und Geschlecht (männlich, weiblich, divers). Religiöse, *race*/ethnische, sexuelle, ableistisch oder klassenspezifische Hintergründe und Herkünfte wurden nicht abgefragt, da unser Teilprojekt nicht das Ziel einer Sozialstrukturanalyse, sondern eine empirisch-ethische bzw. medizinanthropologische Analyse im Sinne einer Dekonstruktion von Bedeutungszuschreibungen, Wirklichkeitsformen und Alltage verfolgt (vgl. BECK 2007: 33, für einen ersten Einstieg siehe die Beiträge in BECK, NIEWÖHNER & KEHL 2008 und BECK, NIEWÖHNER & SØRENSEN 2012).[6] Wie bereits erwähnt, waren eine persönliche Ansprache der Berufsgruppen oder Feldforschungen durch die Pandemie nur bedingt möglich. Gleichzeitig führte die Pandemie auch dazu, dass Menschen mit wenig Technikerfahrung bereit dazu waren, ein (virtuelles) Telefoninterview wahrzunehmen. Das bedeutete jedoch meistens, die Interviews außerhalb ihrer Arbeitszeit von zu Hause aus zu führen. Uns wurde deutlich, dass das Forschen zu Diskriminierungen in medizinischen Feldern einen gewissen Grad an Vertrauen voraussetzt, gerade weil die soziale Kontrolle innerhalb der Berufsgruppen sehr hoch zu sein scheint. Gleichzeitig erfordert die Forschung ein hohes Maß an Flexibilität, zum einen aufgrund der sensiblen Thematik und zum anderen aufgrund der begrenzten Erreichbarkeit der Interviewpartner*innen. Gleichzeitig eröffneten sich durch die digitalen Infrastrukturen wie Video(Telefonie) die Möglichkeit, Gesprächspartner*innen über räumliche Grenzen hinweg zu befragen. Hier schließt die Frage an, wer solche Infrastrukturen bedienen kann, da es Einfluss auf das Sampling hat.

Wir verfolgten sowohl eine *Top-down*-Perspektive über Ärzt*innen und Klinikleitungen als auch eine *Bottom-up*-Perspektive über Community-Vertretungen und (aktivistische) Netzwerke, um Interviewpartner*innen zu rekrutieren. Der Rücklauf war trotz der gezielten Ansprachen von Ärzt*innen, Klinikleitungen und Community-Vertretungen und einer monetären Aufwandsentschädigung eher gering. Die Abgeschlossenheit des Forschungsfeldes zeigte sich daher bereits in der frühen Forschungsphase der Rekrutierung und auch daran, wie die Arbeitswirklichkeiten von Pflegenden und (medizinischen) Fachangestellten aussehen und sich während des Pandemiegeschehens verstärkten. Unsere eigene Positionalität im Forschungsfeld wurde uns deshalb bereits sehr früh vor Augen geführt, die eher von Distanz geprägt war als durch Nähe, obwohl Sabine Wöhlke selbst examinierte Pflegefachkraft ist und über 15 Jahre in diesem Bereich tätig war (vgl. HORNSCHEIDT 2016). Aufgrund der Mehrbelastung durch die Pandemie verschoben sich die Kapazitäten und Prioritäten von im Gesundheitssystem Tätigen. Augenmerk wurde auf die Stabilisierung der gesundheitsspezifischen und medizinischen Infrastrukturen gelegt, weniger auf die Wahrnehmung von wissenschaftlichen Interviewanfragen. Die Zurückhaltung, sich als Gesprächspartner*in zu melden, hängt sicherlich auch damit zusammen, dass das Reflektieren über Diskriminierung von trans*-Kindern und -Jugendlichen innerhalb der eigenen Fachcommunity ein sensibles Thema darstellt, da es auf eigene und fremde Defizite hinweisen bzw. die Gespräche dies potenziell beinhalten könnte. Gruppenzugehörigkeiten und das Berufsverständnis spielten daher ebenso eine Rolle.

Die skizzierten Einschränkungen (Pandemie, Projektdauer, finanzielle und zeitliche Ressourcen) haben deshalb Auswirkungen darauf, dass unser Forschungsprozess nur semi-partizipativ gestaltet werden kann. Sicherlich liegt dies auch an Antragslogiken, die im Projektverlauf wenig Gestaltungsspielraum für spätere Anpassungen zulassen, obwohl die empirische Realität in kollaborativen Arbeitsprozessen oftmals Veränderungen im Forschungsdesign einfordert. Der Projektantrag beinhaltet demnach zwar eine gewisse Offenheit gegenüber den Ergebnissen, allerdings müssen Governancefragen, Zuständigkeiten und die Reichweite des Mitspracherechtes bereits in der Konzeptionalisierung festgelegt werden, was ein Hindernis für spätere Modifizierungen darstellt.

Alle Interviews wurden transkribiert und zum jetzigen Zeitpunkt mithilfe der Software *MAXQDA* inhaltsanalytisch und theoriegeleitet ausgewertet (vgl. MAYRING 2022). Alle Daten wurden pseudonymisiert. Wir arbeiten mit Aliasnamen. Für das Forschungsprojekt liegt ein Ethikvotum der Universitätsmedizin Göttingen vor (2020-162-f-S). Neben der Frage nach der Forschungsethik problematisierten wir ebenso das Forschungsdatenmanagement. So stehen wir vor der Herausforderung, eine große Menge an Tonaufnahmen und Transkriptionen nachhaltig zu sichern, die Zugänge zu regulieren und zu verhindern, dass unbefugte Akteur*innen diese nutzen bzw. Persönlichkeitsprofile rekonstruieren können. Ein längerfristiges Ziel könnte darüber hinaus sein, die Interviews angemessen aufzubereiten und beispielsweise mit Communities zu vergemeinschaften oder die Methode der Fokusgruppe zu nutzen, um die Ergebnisse status- und professionsübergreifend zu diskutieren und zu evaluieren. Denn in der Recherche wurde deutlich, dass eine Vielzahl von Forschungsprojekten zu Transidentität und Diskriminierungen im Gesundheitswesen existieren, diese jedoch spezifische Zielgruppen haben: trans*-Kinder und -Jugendliche selbst, Peergroups, medizinische „Expert*innen", Sorgeberechtigte usw. Zukünftig könnte eine Verknüpfung der verschiedenen Ergebnisse angestrebt werden.

Des Weiteren gilt es, die Selbst- und Fremdregulierungen der Gesprächspartner*innen zu berücksichtigen: Das Medium Interview ist keine neutrale Form der Erzählung, sondern durch eine zeitliche und örtliche Rahmung, narrative Strukturen und Auslassungen gekennzeichnet.

Erfahrungen und Erinnerungen wurden vergessen, verschwiegen oder umgedeutet, gerade auch wenn es um Diskriminierungsformen im eigenen sozialen Nahbereich und in Arbeitskontexten geht. So betonten einige Gesprächspartner*innen zu Beginn des Gesprächs mit Nachdruck, dass sie nicht diskriminieren würden. Dies kann als ein Hinweis für eine fehlende Akzeptanz einer mangelnden Fehlerkultur innerhalb ihrer Profession, als Verweis auf die alltagsmoralische Aufladung des Diskriminierungsbegriffes sowie auf Statusunterschiede im Feld gedeutet werden (vgl. VON DOBENECK & ZINN-THOMAS 2014): Denn einige Gesprächspartner*innen wünschten sich in den Gesprächen eine Rückmeldung über die wissenschaftliche „Verwertbarkeit" ihrer Äußerungen. Auch wenn wir betonten, dass uns ihre lebensweltlichen Perspektiven interessierten, war die Macht des Repräsentationsraumes „Universität" und ihre Praktiken der Wissens- und Wahrheitsproduktion in den Wahrnehmungen omnipräsent. Um den moralischen Vorwurf zu umgehen, näherten wir uns in den Interviews den herausfordernden Situationen innerhalb der Institutionen und Strukturen an, um Handlungsoptionen und -alternativen zu diskutieren und um potenzielle Risiken für eine unbewusste Herabsetzung und Herabwürdigung zu identifizieren.

Diskriminierungen und Stigmatisierungen. Erste Einblicke in die Projektergebnisse

Uns interessieren das Zusammenwirken und die Verflechtungen der individuellen, institutionellen und strukturellen Dimensionen von Diskriminierungen im Arbeitshandeln. Wir fragten

1. nach dem individuellen Pflege-, Betreuungs- und Selbstverständnis,
2. nach biografischen Arbeitserfahrungen und Wissensbeständen (vgl. CARABEZ, PELLEGRINI, MANKOVITZ, ELIASON & DARIOTIS 2015; BROWN, KELLER, BROWNFIELD & LEE 2017) und
3. nach der Rolle der lokalen Versorgungsinfrastrukturen, institutionellen Setzungen und strukturellen Rahmenbedingungen (Gesetze und Bürokratie), zu denen auch die Informations- und Wissensweitergabe innerhalb des Teams und der Institution zählen sowie

die Einbindung von trans*-Kindern und -Jugendlichen in Pflege, Betreuung und Versorgung gehört. Weiterhin wird der Stellenwert des sozialen Netzwerkes deutlich, in das die Pflegenden, (medizinischen) Verwaltungsangestellte, die trans*-Kinder und -Jugendliche und ihre Sorgeberechtigten eingebettet sind.

Eine Bestandsaufnahme der Arbeitsbedingungen in der Pflege und in der (medizinischen) Verwaltung offenbart eine Diskrepanz zwischen den sozial-orientierten Ansprüchen als Pflegende, Betreuende und Versorgende und der Arbeitsrealität, die sich primär durch Missstände auszeichnet und meist ein Gegenpol zu vermittelten Idealzuständen bildet. Diese Diskrepanz, so eine Interpretation, fungiert als Hindernis einer zugewandten und wertschätzenden Pflege. Geschlechtsidentität wird demnach als Zusatzbelastung wahrgenommen, obwohl die beschriebene Pflege- und Versorgungshaltung in den Grundsätzen der Tätigkeit eingeschrieben ist bzw. bereits in den Leitlinien der Berufsgruppen präsent ist. Berücksichtigt werden sollten daher die körperliche und mentale Arbeitsbelastung auf der individuellen Ebene, die strengen Zeitregime, der Schichtdienst, der Fachkräftemangel durch vakante Stellen und Krankheitsausfälle, Machthierarchien und Abhängigkeitsverhältnisse im Team auf der institutionellen Ebene sowie der Stellenschlüssel Patient*in-Pflegefachkraft und die Entlohnungsformen (Geld, Anerkennung und Respekt, Zeitausgleich) auf struktureller und gesellschaftspolitischer Ebene. Insbesondere der Personalmangel ist Gegenstand von politischen Interventionen und Entscheidungen (Tarifverträge, Anpassung des Ausbildungssystems des Stellenschlüssels und der Entlohnungsformen). Er stellt seit mehreren Jahren nicht mehr einen krisenhaften Ausnahmezustand dar, sondern ist „Normalität" geworden auf Stationen, in Kliniken und Ärzt*innenpraxen. Ein Best-Practice-Beispiel, welches in den Interviews mehrfach benannt wurde, ist die *Charité* (Universitätsmedizin Berlin), welches mit Patient*innenführsprecher*innen, (soziale, psychologische und juristische) Beauftragte, Beratungs- und Anlaufstellen für Geschlechtervielfalt, Gleichstellung, Behinderung/chronische Erkrankungen, Antirassismus und -diskriminierung oder (sexualisierte)

Belästigung und Gewalt Handlungsmöglichkeiten und Zuständigkeiten geschaffen hat.

Im Folgenden stelle ich erste Ergebnisse unserer Analyse vor. Aufgrund der Begrenztheit dieses Beitrages erfolgt dies vor allem deskriptiv über Schwerpunktsetzungen. Es lassen sich bis dato vier relevante (Gegen-)Strategien von Diskriminierung, Herabsetzung und Herabwürdigung erkennen, die in der Arbeits- und Alltagspraxis in Erscheinung treten bzw. mehrfach von den Gesprächspartner*innen umschrieben wurden:

1. Das prägnanteste Konfliktfeld, welches in den Gesprächen benannt wurde, stellt das *Misgendering/Deadnaming* in der persönlichen Ansprache und in Schriftdokumenten während der Registrierung, der Behandlung, Pflege und Betreuung dar. Diese Konzepte bezeichnen die aktive aber auch die nicht intentionale, unreflektierte Anrede von trans*-Kindern und -Jugendlichen mit dem bei Geburt zugewiesenen Namen. Gleichzeitig berichten einige Interviewpartner*innen davon, wie sie der Selbstbestimmung von Geschlechtsidentität gerecht werden können, in dem sie zum Beispiel auf den analogen Aktendeckeln oder in den digitalen Infrastrukturen die selbstgewählten Namen ergänzen, auch wenn dies aufgrund der Abrechnungslogiken über die Krankenkassen offiziell nicht erlaubt ist. Mehr noch, einige Interviewpartner*innen entwickelten Strategien wie das gemeinsame Basteln von Türschildern oder Bettzetteln, um sowohl die cis-identen als auch die trans*-Kinder und -Jugendlichen auf die Wirkmächtigkeit von Sprache und ihre wirklichkeitskreierenden Effekte hinzuweisen. Hindernisse stellen teilweise die Vermischung von manuellen und digitalisierten Arbeitsprozessen oder der Brandschutz dar, wenn beispielsweise keine Türschilder angebracht werden dürfen oder das Mobiliar keine Bettzettel zulässt.

2. Des Weiteren wurden in den Gesprächen trans-unsensible und transablehnende Haltungen, Meinungen sowie psycho(patho)logisierende Deutungen des Verhaltens von trans*-Kindern und -Jugendlichen angesprochen, die im Arbeitsalltag präsent sind.[7] So berichten einige Interviewpartner*innen von informellen Gesprächen auf den Fluren, bei Übergaben oder in den Stationszimmern, in denen Kolleg*innen abwertend gesprochen oder das äußere Erscheinungsbild von trans*-Kindern und – Jugendlichen während der sozialen, psychologischen und biologistischen Transition kommentiert wurde. Diese Praktiken wurden als diskriminierend gewertet. Außerdem wurde vereinzelt über Witze und die fehlende Differenzierung darüber gesprochen, welche Bedürfnisse und Zuschreibungskategorien in der pflegerischen und verwaltungsspezifischen Interaktion und Kommunikation mit minderjährigen trans*-Patient*innen überhaupt relevant sind. So wurden Diagnose und Geschlechtsidentität in eine konkrete Kausalitätskette gebracht und den trans*-Kindern und -Jugendlichen, dadurch soziale und psychologische Defizite zugesprochen und sie dadurch entmündigt. Diese Dimension steht symptomatisch für die gesellschaftspolitischen Debatten um Geschlechtsidentität und „Kindeswohl", gerade auch wenn es um die Frage nach Selbst- und Fremdverständnissen geht, wenn zum Beispiel das Kind-Sein dem Trans-Sein gegenüber gestellt oder sie in ihrer Relevanz und Dringlichkeit gegeneinander abgewogen werden (vgl. VROUENRAETS, HARTMAN, HEIN, DE VRIES & MOLEWIJK 2020; HÄDICKE 2022; HÄDICKE, FÖCKER, ROMER & WIESEMANN 2022). Dies trifft meist bei biomedizinischen Geschlechtsangleichungen zu, zum Beispiel die Nutzung von Hormonen, das Abwägen von Konsequenzen und die Zuweisung von spezifischen Rollen (trans*-Person, Kind usw.; vgl. GERRITSE, HARTMAN, ANTONIDES, WENSING-KRUGER, DE VRIES & MOLEWIJK 2018). Diese Argumentation bietet die Gefahr für eine Diskriminierung und Stigmatisierung, gerade weil trans*-Kinder und -Jugendliche dadurch nicht ernst genommen werden bzw. ihren Selbstverständnissen nicht Glauben geschenkt werden.

3. Viele der Interviewpartner*innen waren überzeugt davon, dass sie und ihr Team trans*-Kinder und Jugendliche in ihrem Arbeitsalltag nicht diskriminieren und werteten dies teilweise als einen moralischen Vorwurf, der konträr zu ihrem sozial-orientierten Verständnis als Pflegefachkraft und Verwaltungsangestell-

te*r stand und ihre Vorstellungen von Kollegialität angriff. Wir unterstellen den Akteur*innen in der Pflege, Versorgung und Betreuung nicht, dass sie vermehrt diskriminieren. Viel mehr stellen sich hier Fragen nach unbewussten und nicht intentionalen Herabwürdigungen, Stigmatisierungen und Diskriminierungen (zum Konzept des Unconscious Bias und Transidentität siehe MORRIS, COOPER, RAMESH, TABATABAI, ARCURY, SHINN, IM, JUAREZ & MATTHEWS-JUAREZ 2019). In den Gesprächen wurden Unsicherheiten und Irritationen im Arbeitsalltag umschrieben, die Diskriminierungen bedingen können. Verstärkt werden diese Dynamiken u. a. von einem mangelnden Wissen über Transidentität. In den Schulungsmaßnahmen gilt es daher, das biografische Erfahrungswissen der Berufsgruppe zu stärken und dieses als eine Wissensressource für eine kommunikative Verantwortungsübernahme zu nutzen, gerade auch, um etwaige Unsicherheiten produktiv für eine Sensibilisierung zu nutzen.

Ferner wird in den Gesprächen der Stellenwert des medizinischen Wissens bzw. der medizinischen Deutungshoheiten deutlich. Die Aushandlungen in Ärzt*innenpraxen und auf Stationen in Kliniken bedingen Loyalitätskonflikte, symbolische Kämpfe, Aushandlungen des sozialen Status und Machthierarchien zwischen Ärzt*innen, Angestellten in einem Team sowie den trans*-Patient*innen.

Darüber hinaus spielen die räumlichen Arrangements innerhalb der Stationen und Praxen eine Rolle wie zum Beispiel Toiletten, Warte- und Behandlungszimmer, Zugänge zu Räumen als auch wer welche Rolle innerhalb des Teams übernimmt, gerade auch bei körperlichen Untersuchungen wie das Vermessen von Körpergrößen und Gewicht oder Blutabnahmen.

4. Einige Interviewpartner*innen betonen Gegenstrategien. Sie führten beispielsweise aus, wie sie Diskriminierungen aktiv vorbeugen und entgegenwirken, zum Beispiel, indem sie Risiken und Gefahren von Diskriminierung in spezifischen Betreuungspraktiken und -situationen abwägen. Das heißt, die Interviewpartner*innen artikulierten in den Gesprächen Selbstverständnisse als Lots*innen/

Wissensvermittler*innen und Advokat*innen innerhalb eines Teams auf Station bzw. stationsübergreifend innerhalb der klinischen Institution. Mehr noch, einige Gesprächspartner*innen betonten, wie sie sich Wissen über trans*-Identität in Blogs, Online-Foren, in Podcasts und anderen Sozialen Medien angelesen und anschließend selbstständig vermittelt haben. Dieses Wissen ist jedoch nicht wertneutral, sondern bedarf einer Quellenkritik und der kritischen Einordnung des jeweiligen Mediums und ihrer Formen der Wissensproduktion, -aufbereitung und -rezeption. Deshalb ist aufbereitetes Praxiswissen nach wissenschaftlichen Kriterien, wie wir es generieren werden, umso wichtiger.

Die Interviewpartner*innen wünschten sich Bildungsangebote und Wissensressourcen wie Handzettel, Broschüren und Vermittlungen, um das Thema trans* nachhaltig in ihren Institutionen zu verankern (zum Potenzial siehe OBEDIN-MALIVER, GOLDSMITH, STEWART, WHITE, TRAN, BRENMAN, WELLS, FETTERMAN, GARCIA & LUNN 2011). Es sind gerade diese Form der Wissensvermittlung in den pflegerischen und verwaltungsorientierten Berufsfeldern, die Wissen der heterogenen Zielgruppe gerecht aufbereiten, über Fallbeispiele erklären sowie Handlungsorientierungen und Diskussionsgrundlagen schaffen. Während der Pandemie wurden die arbeits- und tätigkeitsspezifischen Ressourcen auf die Aufrechterhaltung der gesundheitlichen Infrastrukturen gelenkt. Formen der Wissensaneignung durch Schulungen und Weiterbildungen, also konkrete Bildungsangebote, wurden untergeordnet und fielen aus.

In der Diskussion und Evaluation der Ergebnisse wurden erste Widerstände deutlich: Zum einen wurde bejaht, die Individualität von Patient*innen anzuerkennen und ihr gerecht zu werden, zum anderen wurden Bedenken geäußert, die Kommunikations- und Interaktionsformen in der Arbeitsrealität und in den Arbeitsroutinen umsetzen zu können. Dies weißt zum einen darauf hin, zu vermitteln, dass eine Tätigkeit im Gesundheitswesen ohne eine Fehlerkultur nur bedingt möglich ist, zum anderen, dass Diskriminierungskonzepte meist moralisch aufgeladen sind, gerade wenn es Transidentität und minderjährige Personen betrifft.

Des Weiteren dürfen die trans*-Communities nicht außer Acht gelassen werden, wenn es um die Wissensvermittlung geht. Sie sind sehr kleinteilig organisiert, je nach Stadt, Region oder Bundesland. Eine Immersion als Forscher*innen war uns daher nur bedingt möglich. So existieren unterschiedliche Ansprechpartner*innen, die je nach Bedarf in medizinischen, psychologischen/therapeutischen, juristischen und sozialen Belangen zuständig sind. Die Netzwerkbildung innerhalb der Bundesrepublik Deutschland dienen meist der Sichtbarmachung, einer kollektiven Vernetzung und Unterstützung. Sie besitzen unterschiedliche Zielgruppen: trans*-Kinder und -Jugendliche, Erwachsene, Akteur*innen aus dem Gesundheitswesen oder andere Berufsverbände sowie Sorgeberechtigte. Sie bieten Verweisberatungen an und bündeln Anlaufstellen auf ihren Homepages oder positionieren sich zum aktuellen Zeitgeschehen. Zum anderen fungieren sie als soziale Kontrollinstanz innerhalb der Netzwerke und regulieren Zugänge. Ihr Wissen ist produktive Ressource für politische Entscheidungen und Interventionen. Auch für uns haben diese Wissensnetzwerke einen hohen Stellenwert. Unser Ziel, Schulungsmaßnahmen zu entwickeln, knüpft an die Beratungssituationen an. Dies setzt voraus, das generierte Wissen anwendbar zu machen.

Die Netzwerke wirken, so merkten wir es während unserer Forschung, jedoch in sich geschlossen. Sie sind „geschützte Räume". Auch die Einstellung gegenüber dem Wissenschaftssystem fällt teilweise skeptisch aus, da häufig über sie, aber nicht mit ihnen gesprochen wurde. Diese Haltung der Gruppierungen ist historisch bedingt. Im Forschungsfeld um Geschlechtsidentitäten betrifft dies vor allem die Psycho(patho)logisierung und Medikalisierung von Transidentität.

Sichtbarmachen, eingreifen, verändern? Ausblick

Wir haben zu zeigen versucht, wie wir unter Pandemiebedingungen sozial-empirisch geforscht haben, welche Herausforderungen, Potenziale und Grenzen die Rekrutierung von und die Gespräche mit Pflegenden und medizinischen Fach-

und Verwaltungsangestellten mit sich brachte und wie erste Ergebnisse einzuordnen sind. Es lässt sich festhalten, dass sowohl die Tätigkeitsbereiche in der professionellen Pflege, Betreuung und Versorgung auf Stationen in Kliniken und in Ärzt*innenpraxen als auch Transidentität sensibel sind und Eigenlogiken folgen. Die globale Covid-19-Pandemie verstärkte die Arbeitsbelastungen der Pflegenden und medizinischen Fach- und Verwaltungsangestellten im und Zugänge für trans*-Kinder und -Jugendliche zum Gesundheitssystem massiv und zeigte Leerstellen und blinde Flecken in der Forschungspraxis und in der Sichtbarmachung von Diskriminierungen im Gesundheitswesen.[8]

Das Hamburger Teilprojekt lenkt den Blick auf trans*-Kinder und -Jugendliche und individuelle, institutionelle und strukturelle Diskriminierungs- und Stigmatisierungsrisiken in der Gesundheitsversorgung. Sie stellen eine vulnerable Gruppe dar, die sich im Netzwerk zwischen Sorgeberechtigten, Betroffenen- und Communityvertretungen sowie medizinischem Personal positionieren und behaupten müssen. Gleichzeitig sind die Berufsfelder im Gesundheitswesen selbst durch Be- und Überlastungen gekennzeichnet und bedürfen politischer Entscheidungen und Interventionen.

Die von uns herausgearbeiteten Dimensionen zeigen, wie den trans*-Kindern und -Jugendlichen Selbstbestimmung und Handlungsmacht abgesprochen wird, wie ihnen jedoch gleichzeitig eine Schutzbedürftigkeit zugeschrieben wird, die es nicht in Frage zu stellen gilt.

In diesen Bewertungen spielen daher sowohl die Pflege-, Betreuungs- und Versorgungsverständnisse eine Rolle als auch der Anspruch, den Patient*innen mit einem wertschätzenden und individualisierten Umgangsformen entgegenzutreten. Rechtsprechungen und institutionelle Arbeitsabläufe regulieren darüber hinaus individuelle Entscheidungs- und Betreuungsmöglichkeiten.

Weitere Forschung ist notwendig, um die intersektionalen Verflechtungen zu ergründen, die auf trans*-Kinder und -Jugendliche im Gesundheitssystem einwirken und teilweise eine Verstärkung von Diskriminierung und Stigmatisierung begründen. Dies betrifft daher eine geschlechtssensible, barrierearme und inkludierende Pflege und medizinische Verwaltung. Unsere Interviewpartner*innen wünschen mehr Orientierung zum Beispiel durch einen Leitfaden oder Handlungsempfehlung für diesen speziellen Versorgungsbereich, der andererseits einen von vielen weiteren speziellen Pflegesettings darstellt, die es in einer pluralistischen Gesellschaft zu berücksichtigen gilt (siehe auch NIEDER, STRAUSS 2016; LANDESZENTRALE FÜR GESUNDHEITSFÖRDERUNG IN RHEINLAND PFALZ E. V. 2018; SCHUBERT 2021; ÄRZTEZEITUNG 2022).

Wir können als cis-Personen nicht die Sprecher*innenpositionen für trans*-Kinder und -Jugendlichen einnehmen oder gar suggerieren, dass ihre Erfahrungswerte kollektiviert werden können. Als Forscher*innen verstehen wir uns daher teilweise als „Allies", welche die privilegierte Position des Forschungsprojektes nutzen, um die Lebensrealitäten im Gesundheitssystem diskriminierter Akteur*innengruppen sichtbar zu machen – sowohl die trans*-Kinder und -Jugendlichen als auch die Pflegefachkräfte und medizinischen Fach- und Verwaltungsangestellten. Jedoch formulieren wir keine Forderungen auf der (partei-)politischen Ebene wie es beispielsweise die Communities oder Aktivist*innen tun. Im Sinne eines diskriminierungsfreien Gesellschaftsverständnisses bestärkt unser Projekt einen transsensiblen Umgang in Gesundheitsberufen, angestoßen durch Bildungs- und Vermittlungsangebote.

Unser Teilprojekt hat demnach den Anspruch ein Problemfeld, Konflikte und Aushandlungsprozesse nachzuzeichnen, Werte-, Normen- und Moralverständnisse zu hinterfragen und weitere Fragen aufzuwerfen. Es kann daher nur ein erster Schritt in der systematischen Aufbereitung von Wissen über Gesundheitssystem und Geschlechtsidentität sein und einen Perspektivwechsel anstoßen. Hier schließen weitere Desiderata an: Wie sehen die Arbeitswelten von trans*-Pflegefachkräften und (medizinischen) Verwaltungsangestellten auf Klinikstationen in der Bundesrepublik Deutschland aus und wie im (inter)nationalen Vergleich und wie können *Best-Practice*-Beispiele aussehen, die sowohl trans*-Kinder und -Jugendliche als Patient*innen in den Blick nehmen, aber auch trans*-Mitarbeitende in Gesundheitsberufen und ihre Bedürfnisse in Klinikkontexten berücksichtigt?

In den kommenden Monaten entwickeln wir das Schulungs-, Weiterbildungs- und Lehrmaterial und erproben dies in verschiedenen Workshopkontexten u. a. in Münster und Göttingen. Darüber hinaus werden die Ergebnisse aller Teilprojekte zusammengeführt.

Anmerkungen

1 Wir verstehen Geschlecht als soziale und kulturelle Konstruktion und differenzieren zwischen Geschlechtsidentität, -ausdruck, sexueller und romantischer Orientierung sowie die körperlichen Eigenschaften/Bedingungen. Zum einen wollen wir betonen, dass auch innerhalb der Biologie die Zweigeschlechtlichkeit in Frage gestellt wird, zum anderen das Geschlechterbeziehungen und -ordnungen Gewalt, Unrechtserfahrungen und Ausbeutungsverhältnisse bedingen.
2 Der Beitrag basiert auf einem Vortrag beim 19. Arbeitstreffen des Netzwerks Gesundheit und Kultur in der volkskundlichen Forschung der Deutschen Gesellschaft für Empirische Kulturwissenschaft (DGEKW) „Die Ruhe nach dem Sturm? Medikalisierte Alltage in Zeiten der Covid-19-Pandemie" am 07. Juli 2022 (digital).
3 Die Bezeichnung trans* soll die Mehrdimensionalität und Vielschichtigkeit von Selbstverständnissen betonen. Sie schließt Bezeichnungen wie transgeschlechtlich/transident/ transsexuell/transgender mit ein. Die Bezeichnung fungiert als Selbstdefinition und -zuschreibung.
4 Die Pflege, Betreuung und Gesundheitsversorgung von trans*-Patient*innen ist teilweise von lokaler, regionaler, nationaler und globaler Ebene reguliert. So existieren zum Beispiel die *World Professionell Association for Transgender Health (WPATH)* oder Empfehlungen wie *Standards of Care for the Health of Transsexual, Transgender, and Gender Nonconfirming People* oder das *Policy Paper Gesundheit des Bundesverband Trans**.
5 Verbundprojekt TRANS*KIDS. URL: https://trans-kids-studie.de/ueber-uns/ (zuletzt aufgerufen am 23.08.2022).
6 Der große und sehr wichtige Bereich der nicht-institutionalisierten Pflege und Fürsorge wird hier ausgeklammert (für eine kulturwissenschaftliche Perspektive vgl. SEECK 2021).
7 Wir sprechen von „Transfeindlichkeit" und nicht von „Transphobie", da dieser Begriff auf eine Psycho(patho)logisierung von Geschlechtsidentität hinweist. Außerdem möchten wir auf die Vielschichtigkeit des Betroffenheitsbegriffes hinweisen, weil das Konzept zum einen dominante pejorative Bedeutungsdimensionen besitzt, die in der Alltagssprache präsent sind und zum anderen auf die Diskurse über aktive und passive Einflüsse auf Geschlechtsidentität verweist, die aufgrund der Begrenztheit dieses Beitrages nicht diskutiert werden können.
8 Die kulturanthropologische Perspektive auf professionelle Praktiken der Pflege, Betreuung und (Gesundheits-)Versorgung ist ein Ansatz, der sich bereits in den

1970er Jahren herausgebildet hat, natürlich unter den damaligen Bedingungen der akademischen Wissensproduktion und im Sinne der damaligen Fachlogiken und Arbeitsweisen (für einen Einstieg vgl. LEININGER 1970, 1978. Für gegenwärtige Perspektivierungen vgl. WÖHLKE & BENDIX 2017).

Literatur

ALEGRIA, CHRISTINE ARAMBURU 2011. Transgender identity and health care. Implications for psychosocial and physical evaluation. *Journal of the American Academy of Nurse Practicioners* 23, 4: 175–182.

AMELUNG, TILL RANDOLF 2019. Mehr Gesundheit für trans*-Menschen. Wo ist Handlungsbedarf? In NASS, ALEXANDER; RENTZSCH, SILVIA; RÖDENBECK, JOHANNA; DEINBECK, MONIKA & HARTMANN, MELANIE (Hg) *Empowerment und Selbstwirksamkeit von trans* und intergeschlechtlichen Menschen. Geschlechtliche Vielfalt (er)leben. Band II*. Gießen: Psychosozial-Verlag: 81–91.

AMERICAN ACADEMY OF PEDIATRICS 2018. Ensuring comprehensive care and support for transgender and gender-diverse children and adolescents. Policy Paper. *Pediatrics* 142,4. https://publications.aap.org/pediatrics/article/142/4/e20182162/37381/Ensuring-Comprehensive-Care-and-Support-for [26.08.2022].

AMERICAN NURSES ASSOCIATION (ANA) 2018. The nurse's role in addressing discrimination: protecting and promoting inclusive strategies in practice settings, policy, and advocacy. Position Statement. https://www.nursingworld.org/~4ab207/globalassets/practiceandpolicy/nursing-excellence/ana-position-statements/social-causes-and-health-care/the-nurses-role-in-addressing-discrimination.pdf [26.08.2022].

APPENROTH, MAX NICOLAI & VARELA, MARÍA DO MAR CASTRO (Hg) 2019. *Trans & Care. Trans Personen zwischen Selbstsorge, Fürsorge und Versorgung*. Bielefeld: Transcript.

BEAGEN, BRENDA & GOLDBERG, LISA 2012. Nurses' Work With LGBTQ Patients. „They're Just Like Everybody Else, So What's the Difference?" *The Canadian Journal of Nursing Research* 44, 3: 44–63.

BECK, STEFAN 2007. Medicalizing Culture(s) or Culturalizing Medicine(s)? In BURRI, REGULA VALERIE & DUMIT, JOE (Hg) *Medicine as Culture. Instrumental Practices, Technoscientific Knowledge, and New Modes of Life*. London: Routledge: 17–33.

BECK, STEFAN; NIEWÖHNER, JÖRG & KEHL, CHRISTOPH (Hg) 2008. *Wie geht Kultur unter die Haut? Emergente Praxen an der Schnittstelle von Medizin, Lebens- und Sozialwissenschaft*. Bielefeld: Transcript.

BECK, STEFAN; NIEWÖHNER, JÖRG & SØRENSEN, ESTRID (Hg) 2012. *Science and Technology Studies. Eine sozialanthropologische Einführung*. Bielefeld: Transcript.

BÖHM, MAIKA & VOSS, HEINZ-JÜRGEN 2022a. Zur Thematisierung von Trans- und Intergeschlechtlichkeit in medizinisch-therapeutischen, gesundheitsbezogenen und pädagogischen Studiengängen und Berufsausbildungen. *Zeitschrift für Sexualforschung* 35: 5–19.

BROKMEIER, TINA; MUCHA, SANDRA; ROMER, GEORG & FÖCKER, MANUEL 2022. Trans*-Jugendliche und junge Erwachsene im Gesundheitswesen. Eine qualitative Studie über Erfahrungen, Herausforderungen und Wünsche. *Praxis der Kinderpsychologie und Kinderpsychiatrie* 7: o. A.BROWN, CHRIS; KELLER, CHAD; BROWNFIELD, JENNA M. & LEE, REBEKAH 2017. Predicting Trans-Inclusive Attitudes of Undergraduate Nursing Students. *The Journal of Nursing Education* 56, 11: 660–669.

CARABEZ, REBECCA; PELLEGRINI, MARION; MANKOVITZ, ANDREA; ELIASON, MICHELE J. & DARIOTIS, WEI MIN 2015. Nursing students' perceptions of their knowledge of lesbian, gay, bisexual, and transgender issues: effectiveness of a multi-purpose assignment in a public health nursing class. *The Journal of Nursing Education* 541: 50–53.

CICERO, ETHAN C. & PERRY BLACK, BETH 2015. „I Was a Spectacle … A Freak Show at the Circus". A Transgender Person's ED Experience and Implications for Nursing Practice. *Journal of Emergency Nursing* 421: 25–30.DEUTSCHER BUNDESTAG 2022. Zu den Auswirkungen der Coronapandemie auf queere Personen. Studien und weitere Veröffentlichungen. Dokumentation. https://www.bundestag.de/resource/blob/893004/d21396a0adeeaf58f0ddf2bd7b9af00c/WD-9-017-22-Problem-Barrierefreiheit-pdf-data.pdf [26.08.2022].

DÍAZ, DESIREE; MARUCA, ANETTE T.; GONZALEZ, LAURA; STOCKMANN, CHERRILL; HOYT, ERICA & BLACKWELL, CHRISTOPHER W. 2017. Simulation Design: Addressing Care of a Transgender Patient. *Clinical Simulation in Nursing* 13, 9: 452–459.

DU MONT, JANICE; KOSA, SARAH DAISY; SOLOMON, SHIRLEY & MACDONALD, SHEILA 2019. Assessment of nurses' competence to care for sexually assaulted trans persons: a survey of Ontario's Sexual Assault/Domestic Violence Treatment Centres. *BMJ Open* 9, 5. https://bmjopen.bmj.com/content/9/5/e023880 [26.08.2022].

EUROPEAN UNION AGENCY FOR FUNDAMENTAL RIGHTS 2014. Being trans in the European Union. Comparative analysis of EU LGBT survey data. Luxembourg: Publications Office of the European Union. https://fra.europa.eu/sites/default/files/fra-2014-being-trans-eu-comparative-0_en.pdf [26.08.2022].

FIDELINDO, A. LIM & BERNSTEIN, ILYA 2012. Promoting awareness of LGBT issues in aging in a baccalaureate nursing program. *Nursing Education Perspectives* 33, 3: 170–175.

FIDELINDO, A. LIM; BROWN JR., DONALD V. & JONES, HENRIETTA 2013. Lesbian, Gay, Bisexual, and Transgender Health. Fundamentals for Nursing Education. *Journal of Nursing Education* 52, 4: 198–203.

GAJEK, ESTHER 2014. Lernen vom Feld. In BISCHOFF, CHRISTINE; OEHME-JÜNGLING KAROLINE & LEIMGRUBER, WALTER (Hg) *Methoden der Kulturanthropologie*. Bern: Haupt: 53–69.

GERRITSE, KARL; HARTMAN, LAURA; ANTONIDES, MARTE F.; WENSING-KRUGER, ANNELIJN & DE VRIES, ANNELOU L. C. & MOLEWIJK, BERT C. 2018. Moral challenges in transgender care. A thematic analysis based of a focused ethnography. *Archives of Sexual Behavior* 47, 8: 2319–2333.

GÜLDENRING, ANNETTE 2015. Zur Rolle der Medizin und aktuellen Trans*-Transgesundheitsversorgung in Deutschland. In SAUER, ARN THORBE & BUNDESMINISTERIUM FÜR FAMILIE, SENIOREN, FRAUEN UND JUGEND (Hg) *Gutachten. Begrifflichkeiten, Definitionen und disziplinäre Zugänge zu Trans- und Intergeschlechtlichkeiten. Band I*. Bericht. Berlin: BMFSFJ: 31–41.

HÄDICKE, MAXIMILIANE & WIESEMANN, CLAUDIA 2021. Was kann das Konzept der Diskriminierung für die Medizinethik leisten? Eine Analyse. *Ethik in der Medizin* 33, 3: 369–386.

HÄDICKE, MAXIMILIANE 2022. Von Kinderrechten, sozialen Gruppenzugehörigkeiten und Diskriminierungsrisiken in der Medizin. *Frühe Kindheit* 22, 2: 28–34.

HÄDICKE, MAXIMILIANE; FÖCKER, MANUEL; ROMER, GEORG & WIESEMANN, CLAUDIA 2022. Healthcare Professionals' Conflicts when Treating Transgender Youth. Is It Necessary to Prioritize Protection Over Respect? *Cambridge Quarterly of Healthcare Ethics*, o. A.: o. A.

HARAWAY, DONNA 1995. Situiertes Wissen. Die Wissenschaftsfrage im Feminismus und das Privileg einer partialen Perspektive. In DIES. (Hg): *Die Neuerfindung der Natur. Primaten, Cyborgs und Frauen*. Frankfurt am Main: Suhrkamp: 73–97.

HESS, SABINE 1999. Gender- und Transkulturalitätskonzepte. *Anthropolitan:. Kulturanthropologisches Journal* 7: 5–54.

HOPF, CHRISTEL 2019. Qualitative Interviews. Ein Überblick. In FLICK, UWE; VON KARDORFF, ERNST & STEINKE, INES (Hg) *Qualitative Sozialforschung. Ein Handbuch*. 13. Auflage. Reinbek bei Hamburg: Rowohlt: 349–360.

HORNSCHEIDT, LANN 2016. „ABER WIE SOLL ICH DAS DENN MACHEN? INTERDEPENDENKEND FORSCHEN. Methodologische und methodische Handlungsvorschläge." In AK FORSCHUNGSHANDELN (Hg) *Interdependenken! Wie Positionierung und Intersektionalität forschend gestalten?* w_orten & meer: Maintal: 194–214.

HUNTER, JESSICA; BUTLER, CATHERINE & COOPER, KATE 2021. Gender minority stress in trans and gender diverse adolescents and young people. *Clinical Child Psychology and Psychiatry* 26, 4: 1182–1195.

JENNER, CHRISTOPHER O. 2010. Transsexual primary care. *Journal of the American Academy of Nurse Practicioners* 22, 8: 403–408.

KELLETT, PETER & FITTON, CHANTELLE 2017. Supporting transvisibility and gender diversity in nursing practice and education. Embracing cultural safety. *Nursing Inquiry* 24, 1: o. A.

KEEPNEWS, DAVID M 2011. Lesbian, gay, bisexual, and transgender health issues and nursing. Moving toward an agenda. *ANS. Advances in Nursing Science* 3, 2: 163–170.

KNECHT, MICHI 2013. Nach Writing Culture, mit Actor-Network. Ethnografie/ Praxeografie in der Wissenschafts-, Medizin- und Technikforschung. In HESS, SABINE, MOSER, JOHANNES & SCHWERTL, MARIA (Hg) *Europäisch-ethnologisches Forschen. Neue Methoden und Konzepte*. Berlin: Reimer: 79–107.

KRELL, CLAUDIA & OLDEMEIER, KERSTIN 2016. I am what I am. Erfahrungen von lesbischen, schwulen, bisexuellen,

trans* und queeren Jugendlichen in Deutschland. *Gender* 2: 46–64.

LANDESZENTRALE FÜR GESUNDHEITSFÖRDERUNG IN RHEINLAND-PFALZ E. V. 2018. Pflege unterm Regenbogen. Über den Umgang mit homosexuellen, bisexuellen, transidenten und intersexuellen Menschen in der Kranken- und Altenpflege. https://msagd.rlp.de/fileadmin/msagd/Publikationen/Soziales/LZG_Pflege_unterm_Regenbogen_LSBTI_2018_web.pdf [26.08.2022].

LEININGER, MADELEINE 1970. *Nursing and Anthropology. Two Worlds to Blend*. London: Wiley.

——— 1978. *Transcultural Nursing. Concepts, Theories and Practices*. London: Wiley.

LESBEN- UND SCHWULENVERBAND (LSVD) E. V. 2022. Corona. Auswirkungen auf Lesben, Schwule, Bisexuelle, Trans- und Intergeschlechtliche Menschen. https://www.lsvd.de/de/ct/2067-Corona-Auswirkungen-auf-Lesben-Schwule-Bisexuelle-trans-und-intergeschlechtliche-Menschen [01.09.2022].

MAYRING, PHILIPP 2022. Qualitative Inhaltsanalyse. Grundlagen und Techniken. 13. Auflage. Weinheim: Beltz.

MCCAVE, EMILY L.; APTAKER, DENNIS; HARTMANN, KIMBERLY D. & ZUCCONI, REBECCA 2019. Promoting Affirmative Transgender Health Care Practice Within Hospitals. An IPE Standardized Patient Simulation for Graduate Health Care Learners. *MedEdPORTAL. The Journal of Teaching and Learning Resources* 13, 15. https://www.mededportal.org/doi/full/10.15766/mep_2374-8265.10861 [26.08.2022].

MCDOWELL, ALEX & BOWER, KELLY M. 2016. Transgender Health Care for Nurses. An Innovative Approach to Diversifying Nursing Curricula to Address Health Inequities. *The Journal of Nursing Education* 55, 8: 476–479.

MEDINA, CAROLINE; MAHOWALD, LINDSAY; SANTOS, THEE & GURBERG, SHARITA 2021. Protecting and Advancing health care for transgender adult communities. https://www.americanprogress.org/article/protecting-advancing-health-care-transgender-adult-communities/ [26.08.2022].

MERRYFEATHER, LYN & BRUCE, ANNE 2014. The Invisibility of Gender Diversity: Understanding Transgender and Transsexuality in Nursing Literature. *Nursing Forum. An Independent Voice for Nursing* 49, 2: 110–123.

MORRIS, MATTHEW; COOPER, ROBERT L.; RAMESH, ARMANDLA; TABATABAI, MOHAMMAD; ARCURY, THOMAS A.; SHINN, MARYBETH; IM, WANSOO/ JUAREZ, PAUL & MATTHEWS-JUAREZ, PATRICIA 2019. Training to reduce LGBTQ-related bias among medical, nursing, and dental students and providers. A systematic review. *BMC Medical Education* 19, 1, 325. https://bmcmededuc.biomedcentral.com/articles/10.1186/s12909-019-1727-3 [26.08.2022].

MÖLLER, BIRGIT; GÜLDENRING ANNETTE; WIESEMANN, CLAUDIA & ROMER, GEORG 2018. Geschlechtsdysphorie im Kindes- und Jugendalter. Behandlung und Entwicklungsförderung im Spannungsfeld von gesellschaftlichen Kontroversen, Wertewandel und Kindeswohl. *Kinderanalyse* 26, 3: 228–263.

MUCHA, SANDRA; BROKMEIER, TINA; RAREY, FRANZISKA; ROMER, GEORG & FÖCKER, MANUEL 2022 (eingereicht). Transidentität im Kindes- und Jugendalter. Herausforderungen in der Gesundheitsversorgung. *Zeitschrift für Kinder- und Jugendpsychiatrie und Psychotherapie* o. A.: o. A.

——— 2022. Erfahrungen im Gesundheitswesen von Sorgeberechtigten eines Kindes oder Jugendlichen mit Geschlechtsinkongruenz und Geschlechtsdysphorie: Eine qualitative Studie. *Praxis der Kinderpsychologie und Kinderpsychiatrie* 7: o. A.

NÄSER-LATHER, MARION 2021. Von biologischen Tatsachen und komplementären Schöpfungswesen. Geschlechterwissen in ‚wissenschaftlicher‘ Kritik an den Gender Studies. In *Hamburger Journal für Kulturanthropologie (HJK)* 13: 470–180.

NATIONALES MUSTERCURRICULUM KOMMUNIKATIVE KOMPETENZ IN DER PFLEGE (NaKomm) o. A. „Trans* Personen in der Pflege.“ *Homepage Nakomm.ipp.uni-bremen.de.* http://nakomm.ipp.uni-bremen.de/le/trans-personen-in-der-pflege-1-2/ [26.08.2022].

NIEDER, TIMO O. & STRAUSS, BERNHARD 2016. Leitlinienentwicklung in der Transgender-Gesundheitsversorgung. Partizipative Ansätze zwischen Wunsch und Wirklichkeit. SCHOCHOW, MAXIMILIAN; GEHRMANN, SASKIA & STEGER, FLORIAN (Hg) *Inter* und Trans*identitäten. Ethische, soziale und juristische Aspekte*. Gießen: Psychosozial-Verlag: 349–364.

ÄRZTEZEITUNG 2022. Schutz vor Diskriminierung. Hamburger Linke will Förderprogramm für queersensible Pflege. https://www.aerztezeitung.de/Nachrichten/Hamburger-Linke-will-Foerderprogramm-fuer-queer-sensible-Pflege-431375.html [26.08.2022].

OBEDIN-MALIVER, JUNO; GOLDSMITH, ELIZABETH S.; STEWART, LESLIE; WHITE, WILLIAM; TRAN, ERIC; BRENMAN, STEPHANIE; WELLS, MAGGIE; FETTERMAN, DAVID; GARCIA, GABRIEL & LUNN, MITCHELL R. 2011. Lesbian, gay, bisexual, and transgender-related content in undergraduate medical education. *JAMA* 306, 9: 971–977.

ROOD, BRIAN A.; REISNER, SARI L.; SURACE, FRANCISCO I.; PUCKETT, JAE A.; MARONEY, MEREDITH R. & PANTALONE, DAVID W. 2016. Expecting Rejection. Understanding the Minority Stress Experiences of Transgender and Gender-Nonconfirming Individuals. *Transgender Health* 1, 1: 151–164.

ROSA, DANILO F.; CARVALHO, MARCOS V. D. F.; PEREIRA, NAYLA R.; ROCHA, NATALIA T.; NEVES, VANESSA R. & ROSA, ANDERSON D. S. 2019. Nursing Care for the transgender population. Genders from the perspective of professional practice. *Rev. Bras. Enferm.* 72, 1. https://www.scielo.br/j/reben/a/J8GsdDH6ZKb96b8DfdXQfbF/?format=html&lang=en [26.08.2022].

ROWE, DENISE; CHYE, YEOW & O'KEEFE, LOUISE C. 2019. Addressing transgender patients' barriers to access care. *The Nurse Practioner* 44, 6: 30–38.

SCHNEIDER, ERIK & WÖHLKE, SABINE 2022. Würde und Einzigartigkeit respektieren. *Pflegezeitschrift* 75: 48–51.

SCHORRLEPP, MARCEL 2022. trans* Personen fühlen sich in Arztpraxen oft diskriminiert. *MMW. Fortschritte der Medizin* 164: 22–23.

SCHUBERT, LEA 2021. Trans Senior_innen in der Pflege. Ein Leitfaden für Pflegekräfte. https://pflege-professionell.at/

trans-senior_innen-in-der-pflege-ein-leitfaden-fuer-pflegekraefte [26.08.2022].

SZÜCS, DARIA; KÖHLER, ANDREAS; HOLTHAUS, MIKA M.; GÜLDENRING, ANNETTE; BALK, LENA; MOTMANS, JOZ & NIEDER, TIMO O. 2021. Gesundheit und Gesundheitsversorgung von trans Personen während der Covid-19-Pandemie. Eine Online-Querschnittsstudie in deutschsprachigen Ländern. In *Bundesgesundheitsblatt Gesundheitsforschung Gesundheitsschutz* 64, 11: 1452–1462.

SEECK, FRANCIS 2021. *Care trans_formieren. Eine ethnographische Studie zu trans und nicht-binärer Sorgearbeit*. Bielefeld: Transcript.

SHERMAN, ATHENA D.; MCDOWELL, ALEX; CLARK, KRISTEN D.; BALTHAZAR, MONIQUE; KLEPPER, MEREDITH & BOWER, KELLY 2021. Transgender and gender diverse health education for future nurses. Students' knowledge and attitudes. *Nurse Education Today* 97, 104690. https://www.ncbi.nlm.nih.gov/pmc/articles/PMC8049084/ [26.08.2022].

STUCKEY, HEATHER 2013. Three types of interviews. Qualitative research methods in social health: *Journal of Social Health and Diabetes* 1, 2: 56–59.

TEZCAN-GÜNTEKIN, HÜRREM 2020. Diversität und Pflege. Zur Notwendigkeit einer intersektionalen Perspektive in der Pflege. In BUNDESZENTRALE FÜR POLITISCHE BILDUNG (BpB) (Hg): *Pflege. Praxis – Geschichte – Politik*. Bonn: BpB: 250–265.

TOOMEY, RUSSELL B. 2021. Advancing Research on Minority Stress and Resilience in Trans Children and Adolescents in the 21st Century. *Child Development Perspectives* 15, 2: 96–102.

THUMM, DANIEL 2022. *Interaktion mit trans* Patient*innen. Die Pflegebeziehung diskriminierungsfrei gestalten*. Bachelorarbeit. Hamburg: Hochschule für Angewandte Wissenschaft (HAW).

VAN DER DONK, CYRILLA; VAN LANEN, BAS & WRIGHT, MICHAEL T. 2014. *Praxisforschung im Sozial- und Gesundheitswesen*. Göttingen: Hogrefe.

VON DOBENECK, FLORIAN & ZINN-THOMAS, SABINE. 2014. „Statusunterschiede im Forschungsprozess.“ In BISCHOFF, CHRISTINE; OEHME-JÜNGLING KAROLINE & LEIMGRUBER, WALTER (Hg) *Methoden der Kulturanthropologie*. Bern: Haupt: 86–101.

VOSS, HEINZ-JÜRGEN 2021. *Verankerung der Wissens- und Kompetenzentwicklung zu den Themen Trans- und Intergeschlechtlichkeit in den Bildungslehrplänen und Curricula von Ausbildungs- und Studiengängen relevanter Sozial- und Gesundheitsberufe*. Policy Paper. Merseburg: Hochschule Merseburg.

VOSS, HEINZ-JÜRGEN & BÖHM, MAIKA 2022b. Trans*- und Intergeschlechtlichkeit in der Ausbildung [fokussiert auf Pflege]. *Pflegezeitschrift* 6: 44–47.

VROUENRAETS, LIEKE J. J. J.; HARTMAN, LAURA A.; HEIN, IRMA M.; DE VRIES, ANNELOU L. C. & MOLEWIJK, BERT A. C. 2020. Dealing with moral challenges in treatment of transgender children and adolescents. Evaluating the role of moral case deliberation. *Archives of Sexual Behavior* 49: 2619–2634.

WEISS, ILKA CHRISTIN 2019. Umgang mit Trans* in der Pflege. In: NASS, ALEXANDER; RENTZSCH, SILVIA; RÖDENBECK,

Johanna; Deinbeck, Monika & Hartmann, Melanie (Hg) *Empowerment und Selbstwirksamkeit von trans* und intergeschlechtlichen Menschen. Geschlechtliche Vielfalt (er)leben. Band II*. Gießen: Psychosozial-Verlag: 63–81.

Wiesemann, Claudia 2020. Trans-Identität bei Kindern und Jugendlichen. Medizinethische Grundsätze für individuelle Behandlungsentscheidungen. *Praxis der Kinderpsychologie und Kinderpsychiatrie* 69: 517–523.

Wöhlke, Sabine & Wiesemann, Claudia 2016. Moral distress im Pflegealltag und seine Bedeutung für die Implementierung von Advance Care Planning. *Pflegewissenschaft* 5–6, 18: 280–287.

Wöhlke, Sabine & Bendix, Regina 2017. PflegeKultur – Care-Culture. Einblicke in ein Lehrforschungsprojekt, dass Pflege(n) als kulturwissenschaftliche Perspektive beforschte. *Mabuse* 227, 42: 49–52.

Wöhlke, Sabine & Schicktanz, Silke 2019. Research ethics in empirical ethics studies: Case studies and commentaries. *Journal of Empirical Research on Human Research Ethics* 14, 5: 424–427.

Wright, Michael T.; Kilian, Holger & Brandes, Sven 2013. Praxisbasierte Evidenz in der Prävention und Gesundheitsförderung bei sozial Benachteiligten. *Das Gesundheitswesen* 75, 6: 380–385.

Zunner, Brian & Grace, Pamela J. 2012. The Ethical Nursing Care of Transgender Patients. *American Journal of Nursing* 112, 12: 61–64.

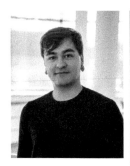

MANUEL BOLZ, M.A., hat Empirische Kulturwissenschaft (vorher: Volkskunde/Kulturanthropologie) und Germanistik an der Universität Hamburg studiert. Er konnte bereits erste Berufserfahrung als studentische/wissenschaftliche Hilfskraft, Tutor, Lehrbeauftragter und studentischer Angestellter am Institut für Empirische Kulturwissenschaft und Germanistik an der Universität Hamburg sowie in der Stabsstelle Gleichstellung und im Zentrum Gender & Diversity (ZGD) sammeln. Er ist Projektassistenz in der Veranstaltungsbetreuung und Vermittlung im Museum am Rothenbaum – Künste und Kulturen der Welt (MARKK) (Elternzeitvertretung) und nimmt in den Jahren 2022/23 ein Forschungsstipendium der Isa Lohmann-Siems Stiftung wahr (Thema: „KörperZeiten. Narrative, Praktiken und Medien"). Des Weiteren arbeite(e) er als wissenschaftlicher Projektmitarbeiter für die Hamburger Behörde für Kultur und Medien (BKM), koordinierte dort die Workshopreihe zur Neu-Kontextualisierung und Dekolonisierung des weltweit größten Bismarck-Denkmal im Alten Elbpark in Hamburg sowie für das medizinanthropologische und empirisch-ethische Hamburger Teilprojekt des Verbundprojektes TRANS*KIDS.

Universität Hamburg, Institut für Empirische Kulturwissenschaft
Edmund-Siemers-Allee 1, ESA W, 20146 Hamburg
manuel.bolz@uni-hamburg.de

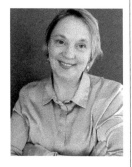

SABINE WÖHLKE, Prof. Dr., hat Kulturanthropologie/Europäische Ethnologie, Geschlechterforschung sowie Medienwissenschaften an der Georg-August-Universität Göttingen studiert. Ihre interdisziplinäre medizinanthropologische, medizinethische Dissertation entstand zum Thema: „Geschenkte Organe? Ethische und kulturelle Herausforderungen bei der familiären Lebendorganspende" (2015 im Campus Verlag erschienen). Von 2008–2019 war Frau Wöhlke am Institut für Ethik und Geschichte der Medizin an der Universitätsmedizin Göttingen als wissenschaftliche Mitarbeiterin beschäftigt. Zudem verfügt sie über eine 16-jährige Berufserfahrung als Krankenpflegerin einer interdisziplinären Intensivstation in der Universitätsklinik Göttingen. Bevor Frau Wöhlke an die HAW wechselte, war sie seit 2019 als Vertretungsprofessorin für den Bereich Pflege am Gesundheitscampus Göttingen tätig. Seit September 2020 ist sie Professorin für Gesundheitswissenschaften und Ethik am Department für Gesundheitswissenschaften der Fakultät Life Science. Sie leitet das Hamburger Teilprojekt des Verbundprojekt TRANS*KIDS.

Hochschule für Angewandte Wissenschaften Hamburg (HAW)
Department Gesundheitswissenschaften
Ulmenliet 20, 21033 Hamburg
sabine.woehlke@haw-hamburg.de

Lehrforum
Teaching Forum

Wir fragen Medizinethnolog*innen nach Texten, Büchern, Filmen oder anderen Medien, die sie in der medizin-anthropologischen Lehre immer wieder gerne einsetzen. Uns interessiert: Warum eignet sich der Text bzw. das Medium besonders gut für die medizinanthropologische Lehre? Was kann an ihm gut aufgezeigt oder diskutiert werden? Zu welchen Einsichten führt dies bei Studierenden? Und inwiefern lässt sich mit den diskutierten Texten bzw. Medien gut weiterdenken?

Wir freuen uns, dass wir mit diesem Anliegen auf so positive Resonanz gestoßen sind und präsentieren hier den vierten Teil einer losen Serie, die kurze essayistische Texte, theoretische Review-Artikel und persönliche Rückblicke auf langjährige Lehrerfahrung einschliesst. Wir hoffen, mit diesen Beiträgen einen längerfristigen Austausch und gegenseitige Inspiration bezüglich medizinanthropologischer Lehre zu ermöglichen. Wer Interesse hat, für eines der folgenden *Curare*-Hefte einen Text auf Deutsch oder Englisch zu schreiben, ist herzlich eingeladen, sich bei der Redaktion zu melden: curare@agem.de.

We ask medical anthropologists about the texts, books, films or other media that they like to use in teaching. We are interested in the following questions: Why is a specific text or medium especially suitable for teaching medical anthropology? What can be demonstrated or discussed particularly well using the text or medium in question?

We are pleased to have received such positive responses and present here the fourth part of a series, which includes short essayistic texts, theoretical review articles and personal reviews of many years of teaching experience. With these contributions, we hope to encourage a long-term exchange and mutual inspiration regarding medical anthropology teaching. Anyone interested in writing a text in German or English for a forthcoming *Curare* issue is welcome to contact the editorial board at curare@agem.de.

Teaching Multiplicities

Von der Arbeit mit multi-medialen Arbeiten

LISA LEHNER & MAGDALENA EITENBERGER

Multimediale Wissenschaft

In den letzten Jahren beschäftigten uns die unterschiedlichsten Themen in unseren gemeinsamen Seminaren: von Medizinethik und Big Pharma über Körperlichkeit und Mensch-Tier-Umwelt-Beziehungen bis hin zum Verhältnis von Medizin und sozialen Ungleichheiten. All unseren Kursen ist kein bestimmtes Medium gemein, wenngleich sie alle aus dem Vollen medizinanthropologischer oder ihr nahestehender Literatur schöpfen. Die für unsere Lehre taktangebenden Medien und Formate sind vielmehr die formoffenen Abschlussarbeiten und -projekte unserer Studierenden selbst. Seit nunmehr drei Jahren leiten wir unsere Studierenden an, ihre Fragestellungen und Analysen in Podcasts, Filmen, Comics, Zines, Interview-Essays, Reportagen und vielem mehr auszuarbeiten. Dieses Jahr erwarten wir auch einen Song. Wenn Studierende entsprechend begleitet werden, die Lernziele erreichen und diese in ihren Abschlussarbeiten umsetzen können, so zeigt unsere Erfahrung, stehen ihnen alle Innovationen und Ausdrucksformen offen.

So erhielten wir in den letzten Jahren Video-Essays zum Leben mit Chronic Fatigue, Comics zu Arbeitsverhältnissen in einer Medikamenten-Verpackungsfabrik, einen Drei-Wissensstufen-Website-Entwurf zu CRISPR-„Genscheren"-Technologie, eine Gegenüberstellung von „disease"- und „illness"-Erfahrungen im Leben mit Depression, Kochbücher und Zines zu Tier-und-Umwelt-Konsumverhalten sowie eine Reihe an Podcast-Episoden mit spannenden Gästen und voll mit berührenden Erfahrungen im Spannungsfeld von Alltag und Gesundheitssystem. Form und Inhalt gehen in diesen studentischen Arbeiten Hand in Hand; Publikum und Empfänger:innen sind mitgedacht; Handgriffe, Schnitte und Farbgebung transportieren Bedeutung auf mehreren Ebenen.

So etwa in einem Comic unter dem Titel *The Crazy Cat Lady*, in dem sich eine Studierende analytisch mit dem in der Popkultur verankerten Klischee einer „Katzenfrau" (engl. „cat lady") beschäftigte, besonders bekannt als Bezeichnung der Eleanor Abernathy in der Fernsehserie *The Simpsons*. Die Cat Lady ist eine (meist ältere) alleinstehende, als weiblich gelesene Person, die eine kennzeichnend enge Beziehung zu ihren vielen Katzen unterhält. Die Abschlussarbeit, die auf den ersten Blick wie eine amüsante Darstellung eines Stereotyps wirken mag, entpuppt sich beim näheren Hinsehen als kritische Auseinandersetzung mit patriarchalen Gesellschaftsstrukturen. Hier werden selbstständige Frauen*, die sich bewusst gegen eine heteronormative partnerschaftliche Beziehung entscheiden, als bemitleidenswert oder – Stigmata rund um psychische Gesundheit bedienend – als „verrückt" bzw. „hysterisch" hingestellt. Die flächige, zweidimensionale Darstellung betont das Naheverhältnis von Katze und Frau, ihre gemeinsame Bedeutung kulturell besetzt und überhöht. Dies ist, wie herausgearbeitet wird, ein „gefährliches Bündnis" in historischer und ähnlich systembedrohender Nähe zu den Hexen, denen ebenfalls Nähe zu Katzen nachgesagt wurde (GEISSELBRECHT 2022). Der 7-seitige Comic funktioniert als Montage unterschiedlicher feministischer, historischer, kultureller und tierrechtlicher Aspekte. Gleichzeitig laden all diese Aspekte in ihrer zeitlosen, nicht-chronologischen Darstellung auf eine immer neu erlebbare Lese- und Gedankenerkundung ein.

Gezielte Wissenschaftskommunikation

Unser didaktisches Ziel, Abschlussarbeiten formatmäßig zu öffnen, besteht darin, Empfänger:innen-zentrierte Kommunikation von Wissenschaft zu erproben. Studierende sehen im ersten Moment und zu Beginn des Semesters die Zahl an Optionen (> 1) für eine Abschlussarbeit zusätzlich zum klassischen akademischen Essay (immer auch eine gute Option) durchwegs posi-

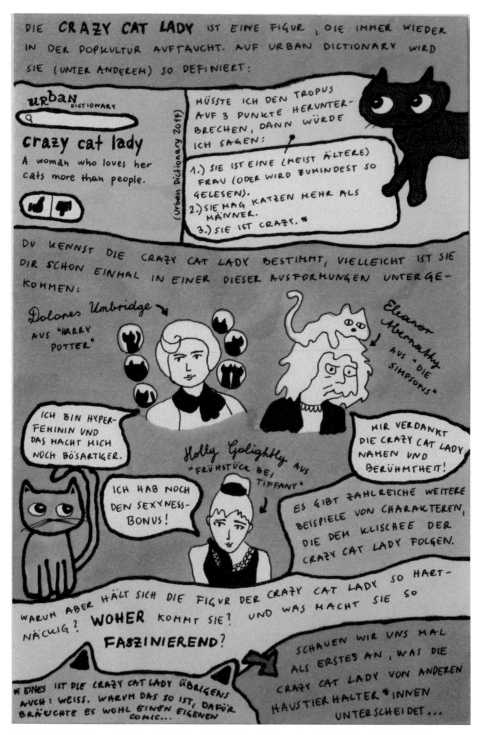

Abb. 1: Beispielseite aus dem Comic *The Crazy Cat Lady* der Studierenden Camilla Geisselbrecht (2022).

tiv und meistens enthusiastisch. Doch im zweiten Moment sehen wir uns stets mit der immer gleichen Frage konfrontiert: „Ist das denn wissenschaftlich?" Oder anders: „*Wie* ist das wissenschaftlich?" Das eigentliche Ziel unserer Übung ist also, gemeinsam mit unseren Studierenden – ganz nebenbei – zu ergründen, was Wissenschaft *sein kann* und was sie *tut*, und gar nicht so sehr, was sie *ist*.

Dadurch beginnen sich unsere Studierenden mit ihrer eigenen Rolle als angehende Wissenschaftler:innen und Analytiker:innen der sozialen Welt zu befassen. Zudem üben sie sich in einer zentralen – und in der Wissenschaft oft fehlenden – Fähigkeit: ihre wissenschaftlichen Erkenntnisse für ein nicht-wissenschaftliches Publikum aufzubereiten. Unter dem Schlagwort „Science Communication" zwar immer wieder gefordert, hat Wissenschaftskommunikation dennoch wenig Bedeutung für wissenschaftliche Karrieren. Legen junge Wissenschaftler:innen Wert darauf, ihre Forschung nicht nur an ihre Kolleg:innen, sondern auch an eine breitere Öffentlichkeit zu tragen, wird das zwar gut geheißen, ersetzt aber in Bewerbungsprozessen kaum klassische Anforderungskriterien wie eine möglichst lange Publikationsliste. Daher setzen wenige Wissenschaftler:innen ein verstärktes Augenmerk auf andere Medien als klassische Texte für wissenschaftliche Journals. Was auf dieser individuellen Ebene mehr als verständlich ist, führt aber gesamtsystemisch dazu, dass Wissenschaft kaum Anreize schafft, über die eigenen Grenzen hinaus zu kommunizieren und einem gesellschaftspolitischen Auftrag der Teilhabe an kleineren oder größeren öffentlichen Diskursen nachzukommen. Wissenschaftler:innen zu sein – das möchten wir unseren Studierenden mitgeben – heißt auch, Verantwortung zu übernehmen. Das ist nicht immer einfach. Schließlich arbeiten wir uns an Fragen der Wertigkeit, der Wichtigkeit, der Positionalität immer wieder selbst ab; lernen auch im Unterricht selbst viel dazu. Der kritische Ansatz der Sozialwissenschaften, die Logiken und Strukturen des sozialen Miteinander zu ergründen, eignet sich im Grundsatz dafür. Diese Art zu denken in andere Medien zu übersetzen bedeutet jedoch, sich ein etwas anderes Handwerkszeug anzueignen – auch wenn die Ansprüche an „gute Wissenschaft" gleich bleiben.

Als Lehrende, die sich interdisziplinär verwurzelt sehen in Medizinanthropologie wie auch in Kommunikationswissenschaften, Politikwissenschaften und Science & Technology Studies (STS), ist für uns beide das *Wie* genauso wichtig wie das *Was*. Mit unseren Studierenden beschäftigt uns nicht nur „Was *ist*?", sondern vielmehr „Wie *wird* (Wissenschaft)?". Vielen – besonders Studierenden im Bachelorstudium, neu an der Universität – wurde noch nie die Position als Mediator:innen wissenschaftlichen Wissens überantwortet. Oft noch sehen sich Studierende als passive Relais des Wissens amorpher, viel zu großer Koryphäen ihrer Disziplin. Der klassische akademische Aufsatz ist für sie sowohl unhinterfragte Form, die Wissen schafft, wie auch Rückzugsort – neutral, im Passiv geschrieben, ein Hort der Fakten.

In „Circulating Reference", einem von BRUNO LATOURS (1999) klassischen Essays zum Wissen-Schaffen, beschreibt er den Weg des Werdens wissenschaftlicher Fakten – von der Expedition zum Diagramm in der Journal-Publikation – und seine Analyse desselben als „deambulatory philosophy" (79): ein Wandern, ein Beschauen, ein detail- und praxisorientiertes Verfolgen. Wir laden unsere Studierenden ein, bewusst zu wandern und zu entdecken – dafür geben wir auch in den Seminareinheiten Zeit. Wissen zu schaffen und dieses zu kommunizieren liegt begründet, so argumentiert auch LATOUR, im Prozess, in seiner Nachvollziehbarkeit, aber auch in seiner Offenheit gegenüber Kritik. Nicht etwa andere von der eigenen Meinung zu überzeugen ist das Merkmal der Wissenschaft, sondern Kommunikation zu eröffnen, Sichtweisen zu erweitern und Dialog zu fördern. Das wollen wir unseren Studierenden vermitteln: Das Fundament von Wissen, Argumentation, Diskussion und Analyse liegt im bewussten *Wie*, nicht im unbewussten *Was*; in der kritischen Auseinandersetzung, nicht im Erscheinungsbild; nicht in der Neutralität, sondern in der Verantwortungsübernahme und -annahme für die Verarbeitung von „situated knowledges" (HARAWAY 1988). Wissenschaftliche – häufig öffentlich finanzierte – Arbeit sollte, so meinen wir, zukünftige Wissens-Schaffer:innen dazu ausbilden, das Angebot einer öffentlichkeitsoffenen Wissenskommunikation machen und Verantwortung dafür übernehmen zu können, was sie tun und was sie sagen.

All das braucht Strukturen: von der Anzahl der Veranstaltungstermine und Deadlines über die reflexive Arbeit mit der Pflicht-„Lektüre" und dem exemplarischen Vorführen möglicher Fragestellungen bis hin zu der offenen Erklärung unseres didaktischen Ziels und Zugangs sowie der gemeinsamen Diskussion der Frage *„Was ist jetzt wirklich Wissenschaft?"* ERIN MANNING & BRIAN MASSUMI (2014) nennen dies die „enabling constraints": die Rahmenbedingungen, die das Feld abstecken und darin Entfaltung erst möglich machen können. Wir versuchen Themenfindung, Fragen(aus)bau und Projektentwicklung zu begleiten mit World Café-Settings, Impulsvorträgen und allerhand praktischen Übungen. Daneben braucht es klare Meilensteine während des laufenden Semesters, einen durchgehenden Austausch und Gruppendiskussionen – das heißt, eine aktive Begleitung der Arbeiten, während diese entstehen, zusätzlich zur in Noten verankerten Beurteilung nach Projektabschluss. Gerade eben in diese Begleitaktivitäten Zeit zu investieren, so zeigt uns die Erfahrung, beeinflusst die Projekte am stärksten. Die Balance zu finden zwischen diesen Aktivitäten und den Inhalten des Seminars fordert uns immer wieder heraus, denn diese Inhalte sind ebenso wichtig.

Medizinanthropologisches Wissen in Form klassischer wissenschaftlicher Zeitschriftenartikel wird hierbei ebenso zu einem Medium wie Graphic Novels à la „The Virus" von MARCIN PONOMAREW & ALEKSANDR BARTOSZKO (2016) zum Leben mit Hepatitis C, die Miniserie des *„You're Wrong About"*-Podcasts zu den Tuskegee Syphilis-Studien (MARSHALL & HOBBES 2020), ein Zeitungsartikel zum Abbau der Statue eines Arztes, dessen Ergebnisse auf Experimenten mit versklavten Frauen beruhen (NEW YORK TIMES 2018), oder Blog-Artikel-Varianten größerer Forschungsprojekte wie VANESSA AGARD-JONES' „Spray" (2014). Wir diskutieren Positionalität der Wissen-Schaffenden, Ansprüche und Anforderungen, Argumente und ihren Aufbau, Publikum und narrative Struktur, Nachteile und Blindspots. Dadurch lernen Studierende in unseren Kursen (vermeintlich) nicht-wissenschaftliche Medien kennen und diese wissenschaftlich zu rezipieren, bevor sie selbst eine multimediale Abschlussarbeit erstellen. Das ist nicht nur für unseren Kurs zentral, sondern bereitet Studierende auch darauf vor, Alltagsmedien – wo passend – in ihr wissenschaftliches Denken und Arbeiten zu integrieren und vor allem kritisch zu diskutieren.

Systemische Bemerkungen

Die Ergebnisse der Arbeiten unserer Studierenden der letzten Jahre sprechen mehrheitlich für sich. 20–40 Studierende optimal zu begleiten ist dennoch immer eine Herausforderung. Die Form kann keinesfalls analytische Schärfe ersetzen – der Anspruch guter und gründlicher wissenschaftlicher Arbeit steht über allem. Wir stützen uns in unseren Kursen darauf, dass die Grundlagen wissenschaftlichen Arbeitens und wissenschaftlicher Methodik in Seminaren mit Kolleg:innen bereits geübt wurden.

Zum Schluss daher noch ein Wort zu den systemischen Bedingungen an den Universitäten der Gegenwart, die unsere Arbeit beeinflussen. Die beschriebenen Kurse und Methoden bestreiten wir im Co-Teaching – eine Praxis, die von Studierenden geschätzt und im Feedback immer wieder als besonders bereichernd hervorgestrichen wird. Co-Teaching gibt die Möglichkeit, innerhalb einer Lehrveranstaltung unterschiedliche didaktische Stile, vielfältige Kompetenzen sowie diverse Forschungs- und Lehrerfahrung zusammenzuführen und für die Lehrgestaltung gezielt einzusetzen. Zudem erlaubt uns Co-Teaching, Projekte in kleineren Untergruppen gezielt angeleitet zu besprechen. Vonseiten des universitären Systems wird Co-Teaching aber oft nicht honoriert und eher als Möglichkeit zur „Arbeitsteilung" beim Lehrveranstaltungsmanagement kontextualisiert. Zumeist und vielerorts gehen damit prekäre Anstellungen externer Wissenschaftler:innen einher. Ohne diese strukturellen Probleme schmälern zu wollen – denn hierfür braucht es dringend politische Lösungen – sind wir dennoch der Meinung, dass innerhalb der gegebenen Rahmenbedingungen kreative Lehransätze möglich sind, die gleichzeitig nicht notwendigerweise das Arbeitspensum für Lehrende erhöhen (müssen).

Literatur

AGARD-JONES, VANESSA 2014. Spray. *Somatosphere*. http://somatosphere.net/2014/spray.html/ [30.12.2022].

GEISSELBRECHT, CAMILLA 2022. The Crazy Cat Lady (Unveröffentlichter Comic).

HARAWAY, DONNA 1988. Situated Knowledges. The Science Question in Feminism and the Privilege of the Partial Perspective. *Feminist Studies* 14, 3: 575–99.

LATOUR, BRUNO 1999. Circulating Reference. Sampling the Soil in the Amazon Forest. In LATOUR, BRUNO *Pandora's Hope: Essays on the Reality of Science Studies*, 24–79. Cambridge: Harvard University Press.

MANNING, ERIN & BRIAN MASSUMI 2014. *Thought in the Act: Passages in the Ecology of Experience*. Minneapolis: University of Minnesota Press.

MARSHALL, SARAH & MICHAEL HOBBES 2020. You're Wrong About. Tuskegee Syphilis Study Part 1: The Lie. https://yourewrongabout.buzzsprout.com/1112270/5330092 [30.12.2020].

NEW YORK TIMES 2018. City Orders Sims Statue Removed From Central Park. https://www.nytimes.com/2018/04/16/nyregion/nyc-sims-statue-central-park-monument.html [30.12.2022].

PONOMAREW, MARCIN & ALEKSANDR BARTOSZKO 2016. The Virus (Comic). http://hepatitiscomics.com/wp-content/uploads/THE_VIRUS_en.pdf [30.12.2022].

LISA LEHNER | BA BA MA MA, ist PhD Candidate am Institut für Science & Technology Studies an der Cornell University, wo sie momentan ihr Dissertationsprojekt zur Heilung von Hepatitis C und der Bedeutung von Wohlfahrtsstaatlichkeit in Österreich abschließt. In ihrer Forschung beschäftigt sie sich allgemein mit Public Health, Marginalisierungsprozessen und sozialer Ungleichheit im Gesundheitssystem sowie wohlfahrtsstaatlichen Strukturen, und macht sich darin ihre Ausbildung in Soziologie, Politikwissenschaft, Medizinanthropologie sowie Wissenschafts- und Technikforschung zu Nutze. In den letzten Jahren arbeitete sie auch als Postgraduate Researcher an der Medizinischen Universität Wien im Rahmen der Horizon 2020 EU-Projekte „SoNAR Global" und „CANCERLESS" sowie als Beraterin bei der Sozialeinrichtung AmberMed und Lektorin an diversen Instituten der Universität Wien und Medizinischen Universität Wien. Ab Mai 2023 startet sie am Institut für Kultur- und Sozialanthropologie der Universität Wien in Zusammenarbeit mit dem Zentrum für Public Health das interdisziplinäre und WWTF-geförderte Forschungsprojekt „Less is More: De-Prescribing Pharmaceuticals for Patient Safety and Sustainable Public Health", in dem sie sich der Verschreibung, Zirkulation und dem Gebrauch von Benzodiazepinen und Antibiotika in Österreich widmen wird.

Cornell University, Department of Science & Technology Studies
303 Morrill Hall, Ithaca, NY 14853, United States
ll723@cornell.edu

MAGDALENA EITENBERGER | Mag.ᵃ Dr.ⁱⁿ BA MA, ist PostDoc in der CeSCoS-Forschungsgruppe zu Zeitgenössischen Solidaritätsstudien am Institut für Politikwissenschaft der Universität Wien tätig. In ihrer Arbeit beschäftigt sie sich mit digitaler Gesundheit und Ethik, Gesundheitstechnologien, Gender und Medizin sowie Gesundheits- und Sozialpolitik. Fachlich ist ihre Forschung in der Politik- und Kommunikationswissenschaft sowie der Wissenschafts- und Technikforschung verankert. In ihrem interdisziplinären Dissertationsprojekt „Technologizing Care in Chronic Illness" befasste sie sich mit politischen Entscheidungsprozessen zu Nutzung, Verteilung und (Nicht-)Finanzierung von Typ 1-Diabetestechnologien im österreichischen Gesundheits- und Sozialsystem. Außerdem unterrichtet sie zu Gesundheitspolitik, Medizinethik und Forschungsmethoden an verschiedenen Instituten der Universität Wien sowie zu Public Health und problemorientiertem Lernen an der Medizinischen Universität Wien. Vor ihrer Zeit am Institut für Politikwissenschaft arbeitete sie als Postgraduate Researcher am Ludwig Boltzmann Institut für Digital Health and Patient Safety und am Institut für Ethik und Recht in der Medizin sowie als Projektmanagerin im Österreichischen Gesundheitsministerium.

Universität Wien, Institut für Politikwissenschaft
Universitätsstraße 7/2, A-1010 Wien
magdalena.eitenberger@univie.ac.at

On Bodies and Our Own Bodies

Care and Vulnerability When Teaching about Death and Loss

MARÍA FERNANDA OLARTE-SIERRA

On a sunny afternoon of mid-March 2022, I stood in front of a group of six students in what was my first teaching experience at the University of Vienna for a course titled *Violence and (dead) bodies. Experiences from (post)conflict scenarios*. Six women, with eager eyes—the only part of their face that I could see since we still were required to wear face masks due to the COVID-19 pandemic that had hit some 24 months before. We all had gone through the experience of living a pandemic that claimed millions of lives. There we stood, six students and I; seven women with distinct socio-cultural and disciplinary backgrounds, and at varying moments and places in our academic trajectory. For most of us, however, this was the first time in two years to be sitting in a classroom with fellow classmates; that we could sit in a group, at a round table in the presence of others—being together—and not looking at each other on a computer screen.

In this text, I reflect on the full spectrum of learning-teaching and focus on the bodily experience of being in the same room where we (students and teacher) become together and leave transformed. I argue that teaching and learning about death and dying in a violent context requires coming together to expose and share our vulnerabilities. This, because in order to make sense of brutal violence without minimising it or essentialising it, we need to allow ourselves to be vulnerable: to acknowledge that we know and understand through and with our bodies. Accepting being vulnerable together enables space for mutual care where we can support each other. Through such vulnerability, we can acknowledge our emotions, recognise our embodiments and reflect on how we each relate to and understand dying a violent death. Together we can explore how, through and with our bodies, we shape the questions we raise about dying in a violent context and also how we grapple with these issues.

Understanding teaching-learning as a bodily experience implies rethinking the format, setting, and methodology of the themes and topics we address. It requires us, as teachers, not only to secure safe spaces where students feel comfortable expressing themselves but also not to take for granted the historical classroom setting (as problematic as traditional forms of learning might be). Additionally, it calls for ensuring the possibility of allowing silence as a form of expression and being present, since emotions are not always easily put into words, for making sense of acts of brutal violence tends to leave some of us speechless. Hence, this is an invitation to rethink the teacher-student binomial in terms of our responsibility to our students to care for them when we address grief and loss (KRYSTALLI 2021). That is to say, to take care when we open up spaces for mutual learning when considering *topics that break our hearts,* paraphrasing RUTH BEHAR (1996).

Affective teaching and learning with and through the body

For this course, we were set to attend to the (dead) body in contexts of mass violence and war around the world. For seven sessions we would address and discuss both the materiality and the power—symbolic and political—of dead bodies. We would dive deep into the nastiness of violence and the marks that it leaves on bodies and the social fabric of a community. We would tackle how and why not all dead bodies are equal since not all people are equally targeted by crime and violence. Matters of race, gender, socio-economic status, ethnicity, ideology, religion, and appearance were all elements to be discussed in our class. The body was to be at the centre of our discussions. Constantly present. We had to acknowledge that before a body was a corpse, it was a person. We had to recognize that a "body count" disregards the life and death of real people and serves as an easy escape route to avoid facing the pain, desolation, and fear that violent death implies. Thus, we were set to be uncomfortable for seven sessions while we faced death and dead bodies. That afternoon in March, sitting with those six students, and still being in the healing process of vicarious trauma due to my research on forensic experts' knowledge practices in Colombia, a country with a long and on-going history of violence (OLARTE-SIERRA 2022), I opened the space to dwell with heart-breaking and conceptually challenging discussions of death and dead bodies in the communal presence of in-person very alive students.

As a feminist, I am aware of the role that affect and emotion have in knowledge production (cp. AHMED 2004) and I not only acknowledge this in my research practice (OLARTE-SIERRA 2019), I actively try to transmit it to my students. However, it was not until this course on violence and (dead) bodies that I engaged in practices—inside the classroom—to attend to how we (both individually and as a group) were feeling and how those feelings shaped the discussions we had and the questions we asked in the classroom space. This was particularly tangible in the third session; a session on "gender and death". The core of the discussion and the readings the students had to prepare were on femicide. The idea was that a student presented the case of gendered bodies of refugees, on the one hand, and on soldiers and casualties in the context of the Ukraine-Russia war that had recently started, on the other. To integrate the pre-class readings and the student's presentation, I had planned to address the challenges of forensic identification of the remains of trans people (especially when skeletal) in the Colombian armed conflict. Then, have a discussion and let the students raise questions or make comments, as we had done in the two previous classes. However, this was not how the class unfolded, it was not as straightforward.

I arrived at class shaken. For me, re-reading the literature for that day was challenging. I had to stop a couple of times to take a breath and a walk. The description of the marks that femicide leaves on women's bodies, the level of apathy these crimes often produce in the general public, and my embodied fear as a woman—and so this could happen to me—were elements that made my reading difficult. When entering the classroom, the students were unusually quiet,

only a few were talking and discussing cases of femicide that they were aware of. I opened the session by asking the women how they felt. After a short silence, I rephrased my question, "how did the readings make you feel?" Silence again. After a couple of minutes in silence and elusive glances, I embraced the responsibility of sharing, which is never easy—not for me, anyway. I talked about my need for breaks while reading and that the images described by the authors came so vividly into my head that I could imagine the suffering of the victims, their mangled bodies, and the cries of their mothers and fathers and friends. I mentioned that my working so closely with violence in Colombia had produced a kind of sensitivity that made what I read translate to me physically—to my body. I spoke about how this work has negatively affected my mental health as well. I also said that I find it problematic that some forms of writing about suffering actually revictimize and essentialise victims and risks reducing their entire existence to the suffering they endured and all that revolved around their death and dying. I finished by saying that despite my pain, I believe that we need to address these topics, we must look directly at violence and death, regardless of our urge to look away because the suffering of others in war ridden or mass violence contexts affects us all as fellow human beings. As researchers we can provide the nuance and greater context and considerations of human lives that does not limit people to their experiences of suffering, death or dying.

The motivation for asking and initiating reflection with my students was part of my own process of healing. I knew all too well that violence, albeit distant and through texts and testimony can have a devastating effect on our bodies and minds. After I finished speaking, the students started sharing and we engaged in a session-long conversation in which we not only referred to the literature but also to how speaking of death, bodies, and violence made us feel in general. As each of us spoke, the others listened attentively. I encouraged questions, but highlighted that if any questions came up, they needed to be posed compassionately even if students disagreed with one another. For me, this was a way of ensuring that we kept an analytical body-mind while providing a safe space to care for and respect the group and each individual. Among the emotions students referred to were despair, fear, anger, and disgust as they found disturbing some of the cases we discussed. As a group, we talked about how we could write about and report issues and topics like these, without traumatising our audiences and revictimizing the victims or avoid addressing these poignant issues. We spoke about how to address victims of violence in ways that do not reproduce the violence but rather effectively communicate our concerns.

From that session onward, we devoted a portion of each session to address how we felt both with the day's topic and the general theme of the course. Addressing our emotions (i. e., how the texts made us feel) allowed us to acknowledge our embodiments. That is, it enabled us to recognize the centrality that our bodies have when we are confronted with any form of knowledge making—whether we are aware of it or not (AHMED 2004; LÓPEZ 2014). Putting forward our embodiments shed light on how we felt with a given session or the course in general. Thus, we were made aware of how our own experiences, emotions, feelings and reactions to death and dead bodies were shifting as a result of participating in the course and discussions in our shared space. We talked about how placing the body of those who died a violent death on centre stage gave the violence we were studying a new nuance, made it tangible, difficult to ignore. This, in turn, required that we search for other words to talk about pain and suffering in ways that convey its matter-of-factness and does not minimise it. We found the value of silence since, on occasion, it was more eloquent than words – for words could not fully express how we felt and what we were thinking. Reflecting on the bodies that suffered the violence and on our own bodies as sites of knowledge production through intellect and affect shaped the experience of our course and our overall relationship to how violence and suffering are referred and documented in academia.

A need for closeness, silence and trust

When I planned this course, I did not anticipate how it would develop. I did foresee that it would be a challenging course for students and for me due to the topic. I was aware of the need for caution regarding my students' and my own emotional well-being. However, I had never expected it to be so hard and beautiful and inspiring—all at the same time. Also, I did not know what to expect from my students, since this was the first time I had taught at the University of Vienna, and was unfamiliar with the kind of engagement students are willing to have as individuals and as a group. Today, in hindsight, I can say that we were a fortunate bunch of seven women who realised we could trust the silences and the presence of the other six in the safe space of a classroom. We could share parts of our own vulnerabilities and jointly go through a learning experience that shaped us all. For me, as a teacher, I learnt to recognise the silence that fills a classroom as an eloquent and welcomed companion. I grew ever more comfortable allowing students the time to think (and feel) before participating, thus, giving them a chance to fully inhabit our collective silence.

We were also a fortunate bunch, because we could have this learning experience while sharing the same physical space. We could be together and make eye contact or direct a smile (albeit behind a face mask) or talk to a classmate in close proximity to one another or share a coffee break. We could hear and feel others' laughter and silence as well as our own resonating in the classroom and not through speakers on our computers. Having put the body centre-stage while addressing life and death in violent contexts required us to acknowledge our own bodies. The COVID-19 pandemic reminded us of our own vulnerability and the Russian war on Ukraine did not let us forget the fragility of life. This course and our being and becoming together was a gentle reminder that life is lived moment by moment. It allowed us—through our losses, fears and expectations—to understand that loss helps to tune inquiry and calibrate responses, which "can inform the 'mmm', the sound of empathy" (KRYSTALLI 2021: 43). That this course and how it occurred reminded us of the power of care and support in whatever form they may take, which for us was a classroom on the 4th floor at the New Institute Building (NIG) of the University of Vienna in the summer semester of 2022.

Final remarks

Following BEHAR's (1996) insight about vulnerable writing, I see that opening a space to be vulnerable together brought about predicaments that I had not anticipated as a teacher (i.e., thick silences, students' discomfort with some topics and forms of writing present in the reading material for the course, and the open acknowledgement of fear and pain). However, this enriched our theoretical discussions and allowed us to nurture the complexity that knowing with and through the body brings. BEHAR says: "this anthropology [of pain and suffering] isn't for the soft-hearted" (1996: 24), and we, together, found our own strengths through vulnerability while we cared for each other by supporting one another in the shared space of a classroom, respecting each other's rhythms, voices, laughter, questions, and silences.

To close this text, I turn once again to KRYSTALLI's words when she says: "feminism is not merely about a series of terrible stories of [...] violence, but also a register of care and a vocabulary of joy" (2021: 43). Care clearly materialised in the classroom in the forms I have shared above. Joy, however, was more elusive. Yet, joy was there as a river that ran deep throughout the course. As a final assignment, I asked each student to write a reflection on what they had learnt in our course and what they took away for future experiences (whether academic or not). The students mentioned the course dynamics, the centrality we gave to the body, the space we opened for connection, to address our emotions and our embodiments; and the safety to speak and be heard. I interpret all these as a form of joy. The kind of joy that wholesome experiences of learning and being together produce. The joy of acknowledging our commitments, expectations, questions (not always answered), and the possibility of being together, supporting one another. The joy of knowing oneself cared for while also caring for others.

References

AHMED, SARA 2004. *The Cultural Politics of Emotion*. Edinburgh: Edinburgh University Press.

BEHAR, RUTH 1996. *The Vulnerable Observer. Anthropology that breaks your heart*. Boston: Beacon Press.

KRYSTALLI, ROXANI 2021. Of loss and light: teaching in the time of grief. *Journal of Narrative Politics* 8, 1: 41–44.

LÓPEZ, HELENA 2014. Emociones, Afectividad, Feminismo. In GARCÍA ANDRADE, ADRIANA & SABIDO RAMOS, OLGA (eds) *Cuerpo y afectividad en la sociedad contemporánea. Algunas rutas del amor y la experiencia sensible en las ciencias sociales*. Ciudad de México: Universidad Autónoma Metropolitana: 257–276.

OLARTE-SIERRA, MARÍA FERNANDA 2019. Of flesh and bone: emotional and affective ethnography of forensic anthropology practices amidst an armed conflict. *Tapuya: Latin American Science, Technology and Society* 2, 1: 77–93.

OLARTE-SIERRA, MARÍA FERNANDA 2022. (Un)Doing the Colombian armed conflict: forensic knowledge, contradicting bodies, unsettling stories. *Social Anthropology/Anthropologie sociale* 30, 3: 19–37.

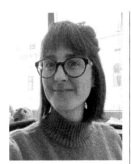

MARÍA FERNANDA OLARTE-SIERRA is a medical anthropologist and an anthropologist of science with a focus on ethnographic research. She addresses interactions of health, technology, and the body in highly bio-medicalized and technological contexts in Latin America. She recently finished a Marie Skłodowska-Curie fellow at the University of Amsterdam with a project that addresses the role of judicial and humanitarian forensic knowledge in co-producing collective accounts of violence in Colombia. Currently, she is a Postdoctoral Researcher at the University of Vienna, in the Institute of Social and Cultural Anthropology in the group of Medical Anthropology and Global Health, where she works on the search for forcibly disappeared persons conducted by people who are living in exile as practices of collective care and sites of reconciliation in war-ridden contexts in Latin America.

University of Vienna
Medical Anthropology & Global Health|Institute for Cultural and Social Anthropology
Neues Institutsgebäude (NIG). Universitätsstraße 7 1010 Vienna, Austria
mafe.olarte-sierra@univie.ac.at

Visual Expressions of Health, Illness and Healing

Bericht zur 34. jährlichen Fachtagung der Arbeitsgemeinschaft Ethnologie und Medizin (AGEM) in Kooperation mit der Österreichischen Ethnomedizinischen Gesellschaft (ÖEG) und dem Weltmuseum in Wien, 2.–4. Juni 2022

HELMAR KURZ & KATHARINA SABERNIG

Die diesjährige AGEM-Jahrestagung wurde unter dem Titel „Visual Expressions of Health, Illness and Healing" in Kooperation mit der Österreichischen Ethnomedizinischen Gesellschaft (ÖEG) und dem Weltmuseum Wien von Katharina Sabernig, Doris Burtscher und Ruth Kutalek organisiert. Thematisch verstand sich die AGEM-Konferenz 2022 als eine Fortsetzung der Konferenz „Ästhetiken des Heilens: Arbeit mit den Sinnen in therapeutischen Kontexten", die 2019 in Münster stattfand. Bei der diesjährigen Tagung standen visuelle Ausdrucksformen von Krankheit und Gesundheit im Kontext klinischer Arbeit und Ausbildung, gesellschaftlicher Sichtbarkeit sowie subjektiver Wahrnehmung im Fokus. Die Konferenz war inter- und transdisziplinär ausgerichtet, mit einem Schwerpunkt auf visueller Medizinanthropologie und den transkulturellen medizinischen Geisteswissenschaften. Eingeladen waren ForscherInnen, KünstlerInnen, KuratorInnen, MedizinerInnen sowie PatientInnen und deren Angehörige, um sich mit ihrer Erfahrung und ihrem Fachwissen einzubringen. Ein weiteres Ziel der Organisatorinnen war es, die Konferenz auch als eine Hommage an Prof. Armin Prinz (1945–2018) auszurichten. Der Arzt und Anthropologe war der erste Professor für Medizinische Anthropologie (Ethnomedizin) in Österreich und Spezialist für visuelle Medizinanthropologie. Er gründete die Österreichische Ethnomedizinische Gesellschaft und legte eine umfangreiche Sammlung ethnomedizinischer Objekte und Bilder an, die 2017 dem Weltmuseum Wien als Schenkung übergeben wurde. Die Tagungssprache war Englisch, was den internationalen TeilnehmerInnen aus Kanada, den Vereinigten Staaten sowie sechs europäischen Ländern entgegenkam. Die Veranstaltung fand in Präsenz statt.

Eröffnet wurde die Veranstaltung am ersten Konferenztag durch den Direktor des Weltmuseums JONATHAN FINE, der in seiner Begrüßungsrede die große Bedeutung einer interkulturellen Betrachtung von medizinischen Themen in Museen und dem öffentlichen Raum betonte. KATHARINA SABERNIG entrichtete Grußworte von Professor Emeritus RICHARD RALSTON (University of Wisconsin-Madison), ehemaliger Gastprofessor in Wien, und EKKEHARD SCHRÖDER, der die lange Tradition der gegenseitigen freundschaftlichen Förderung von ÖEG und AGEM betonte. Anschließend reflektierte RUTH KUTALEK (Medizinische Universität Wien, AT) den ungewöhnlichen Werdegang von Prof. Armin Prinz und sein unermüdliches Interesse, seine beiden Professionen als Notarzt am Flughafen und Sozialanthropologe an der Universität zu vereinen. Um den Blick der Studierenden für die medizinischen oder sozialen Aspekte von Leidenszuständen zu öffnen, richtete er sein besonderes Augenmerk auf die visuelle Anthropologie in all ihren Formen: Foto, Film und später die Sammlung von Bildern afrikanischer KünstlerInnen. In der anschließenden Diskussion wurde seine Tätigkeit als Arzt und Anthropologe in Afrika erörtert und auch seine mikrobiologischen Studien vor Ort beleuchtet. Darauf folgte die Eröffnung der Ausstellung „Schenkung Österreichische Ethnomedizinische Gesellschaft – Eine Auswahl von Populärmalereien aus Kinshasa, Demokratischen Republik Kongo" (2. Juni bis 1. November 2022) durch die Kuratorin für die Sammlungen Afrika südlich der Sahara, NADJA HAUMBERGER (Weltmuseum Wien, AT). Die Präsentation der Bilder fand mitsamt einer Erklärung zur Geschichte der ethnomedizinischen Sammlung im „Korridor des Staunens" (Galleries of Marvel) statt.

Der weitere Tag illustrierte Themen aus Afrika und Amerika im Kontext von Rassismus, Kolonialismus und kommunaler Gesundheitsprojekte mit Hilfe von Narrativen. Die erste Promovendin von Armin Prinz, DORIS BURTSCHER (Ärzte ohne

Grenzen, AT) zeigte, wie PatientInnen und deren UnterstützerInnen ihre Erfahrungen mit der Behandlung resistenter Tuberkulose im ländlichen Eswatini schildern: mittels der visuellen Darstellungstechnik PhotoVoice, durch Interviews und Gruppendiskussionen. Die emotionale Unterstützung und Betreuung weit über die klinische Problematik hinaus wurde als positiv empfunden, während Bedenken hinsichtlich wirtschaftlicher Herausforderungen und das Infektionsrisiko für die Familien und die Community Treatment Supporters (CTS) als problematisch bewertet wurden. In der anschließenden Diskussion wurde auch hinterfragt, ob die CTS dadurch mit gesellschaftlicher Ausgrenzung konfrontiert waren.

Danach erläuterte MEGAN A. CARNEY (University of Arizona, US) lebensbejahende Narrative des Wohlbefindens von zwanzig afroamerikanischen EinwohnerInnen aus Tucson (Arizona), wodurch Gesundheitsportale als Gegenmittel zu institutionellen Strukturen gebildet werden können. Es stellte sich demnach heraus, dass die Kartographie von Orten für die Festigung von Zugehörigkeitsgefühlen von großer Bedeutung ist, um institutionell gewachsenen Strukturen mit rassistisch motivierten räumlichen Logiken zu begegnen.

JUAN CARLOS RODRIGUEZ CAMACHO (University of New Brunswick, CA) präsentierte ein Kunstprojekt, in dem individuelle und gemeinschaftliche visuelle Kunsterfahrung dahingehend untersucht wurde, inwieweit indigene und nichtindigene Vorstellungen von Wohlbefinden ineinandergreifen. Die individuelle und gemeinschaftliche Erfahrung wurde in einem Kurs „Teaching in Cultural Context" (Unterricht im kulturellen Kontext für Lehrkräfte im Vorbereitungsdienst) ermittelt. Dabei wurden Kunst- und Heilungsnarrative in 27 Dreiecken dargestellt, die anschließend in einer Installation co-konstruiert werden. Die angeregte Diskussion um gemeinsame Kunsterfahrung auf Basis von Narrativen berührte auch sensorisch-emotionale Faktoren in Zusammenhang mit visueller Erfahrung von Kultur und Heilung.

Im zweiten Panel stand Gezeigtes im Gegensatz zu Nichtgezeigtem (und umgekehrt). BERND BRABEC DE MORI (Universität Innsbruck, AT) präsentierte die Visualisierung des Unsichtbaren, indem das Konzept des „Ayahuasca-Schamanismus" im westlichen Amazonasgebiet als rituelle

Heilung in Mustern, Gemälden und Filmen veranschaulicht wurde. Traditionell findet menschliche Interaktion mit Tieren, Pflanzen oder Geistern in auditiven Mitteln wie Liedern, Gesängen, Anrufungen und Formeln ihren Ausdruck. Im Kontext der Verschiebung vom Auditiven hin zum Visuellen drehte sich die anschließende Diskussion überwiegend um die Chancen und Probleme einer zunehmenden Kommerzialisierung der „Ayahuasca-Kultur".

Mit der Frage der kuratorischen Verantwortung in einem dekolonialen Umfeld beschäftigte SARAH BÖLLINGER (Universität Bayreuth, DE) in ihrem Beitrag „Glücklose Köpfe", der sich mit der Entstehungsgeschichte von rund 600 Bildern beschäftigte, die von zwölf Patienten und Patientinnen im Lantoro Mental Asylum im Rahmen eines Projektes des deutschen Kunstliebhabers Ulli Beier und seiner ersten Frau, der österreichischen Künstlerin Susanne Wenger, gemalt wurden. Dabei wurde nicht nur der künstlerische Wert der Bilder aufgezeigt, sondern hinterfragt, wie mit Kunst von Menschen in (psychischen) Ausnahmesituationen respektvoll umgegangen werden kann.

Der zweite Konferenztag widmete sich im ersten Panel zunächst der Bedeutung von Piktogrammen und medizinischen Comics. EBERHARD WOLFF (Universitäten Basel und Zürich, CH) fragte nach der Rolle von Piktogrammen im Kontext von Kontrollregimen während der Coronapandemie, innerhalb derer sich medizinische und legale Sphären durchdringen. Er argumentierte, dass sich Status- und Zugangsregelungen in Form von Visualisierungen während der Pandemie hin zu einer „Ticketisierung" entwickelten. In der Diskussion ergab sich die Frage, wie dies Menschen langfristig beeinflussen wird.

Im Anschluss stellten MARTINA CONSOLINI (Universität Bologna, IT) und SARA VALLERANI (Universität Roma Tre, IT) ihr Projekt eines Comics vor, der sich mit der Frage des Rechts auf Gesundheit auseinandersetzt. Diese Frage erschien den Autorinnen während der Pandemie stärker an Gewicht zu gewinnen als zuvor. Mit Bezug auf die historische Person der Käthe Kollwitz nennen sie sich „Käthe Collective" und entwickelten während des Lockdowns 2020 die Idee, eine breite Definition von Gesundheit mit medizinischen und sozialen Aspekten zu unterfüttern, welche auch die Ungleichheit beim Zugang zu Gesundheitsressourcen betreffen. Mit dem Ziel, sowohl PatientInnen als auch Behandelnde einfach verständlich zu informieren, wurde das Werk 2021 online und 2022 als Buch veröffentlicht; englische, französische und spanische Übersetzungen sowie ein Hörbuch werden aktuell bearbeitet.

Der dritte Beitrag von RUTH KOBLIZEK (Medizinische Universität Wien, AT, in Kooperation mit Ruth Kutalek, Andrea Praschinger, Eva Katharina Masel) widmete sich ebenfalls medizinischen Comics, allerdings insbesondere als Reflexionsmöglichkeit für MedizinerInnen in der Ausbildung, d. h. indem sie durch Comics für schwer vermittelbare Themen sensibilisiert werden oder ihre Erfahrungen bildlich darstellen und teilen. In der Diskussion wurde kritisch hinterfragt, ob sich Comics zur Kommunikation unter Professionellen und zur Darstellung komplexer Inhalte eignen. Ein Ansatz, das Vorurteil der Unwissenschaftlichkeit zu vermeiden, könnte die Suche nach einem Alternativbegriff für „Comic" sein.

Auch das zweite Panel widmete sich der Macht des Bildes. ANNA GELDERMANN (Universität Köln, DE, in Kooperation mit Saskia Jünger) untersuchte visuelle Repräsentationen von Gesundheitsinformationen im Internet und wie diese Menschen beeinflussen bzw. wie sie sich innerhalb der Fülle unterschiedlich gearteter Informationen zurechtfinden. An Beispielen von Menopause-Produkten diskutierte sie Habitualisierung und Sozialisierung von Diskursen durch den Einsatz von Bildern in der Kommunikation mit Zielgruppen. In der Diskussion wurde weiter erörtert, wie menschliches Gesundheitsverhalten beeinflusst und kontrolliert wird und wie man mit der Problematik der Desinformation bzw. Sicherheit umgehen kann.

Auch EVA-MARIA KNOLL (Österreichische Akademie der Wissenschaften, AT) beschäftigte sich mit bildlichen Aufklärungspotentialen im Kontext des Designprozesses einer medizinischen Broschüre zur Sichelzellkrankheit, welche die Kommunikation zwischen Eltern und ihren Kindern zu erleichtern sucht. Als Beispiel nannte sie eine Familie mit Migrationshintergrund, der die bildliche Kommunikation komplexer Inhalte sehr geholfen hat, eigenständig Entschei-

dungen zu treffen. Die anschließende Diskussion widmete sich den Fragen, in welchem Alter man was wie kommunizieren sollte und wie mit lokalen Bedeutungen (gerade im Migrationskontext) umzugehen sei. Weiterhin wurde auch das Potential für andere Gesundheitskontexte, z. B. HIV, erörtert.

Das dritte Panel vereinte sehr unterschiedliche Beiträge. PAUL DIEPPE (Universität Exeter, GB, in Kooperation mit Natalie Harriman, Sarah Goldingay, Ayesha Nathoo, Emmylou Rahtz, Sara Warber) beschäftigte sich mit dem Konzept des „Heilens" in der westlichen biomedizinischen Praxis. Er bezog sich zunächst auf ein Projekt, welches er schon auf der AGEM-Tagung 2019 vorstellte und innerhalb dessen er zunächst PatientInnen in einem Krankenhaus Bilder malen ließ, was sie unter Heilung verstehen, und später die Reaktion von TherapeutInnen und BesucherInnen auf die ausgestellten Werke festhielt. In einem rezenten Projekt während des britischen Green Man Festivals verteilte er geschnitzte hölzerne Herzen an Besucher, in denen sie anonym Botschaften hinterlegen konnten, „was sie auf dem Herzen haben", die hinterher ausgestellt und diskutiert werden konnten. Er beobachtete dabei enormes kathartisches und heilendes Potential bzgl. persönlicher Sorgen und Probleme durch das Verständnis innerer Konflikte und deren visuelle Kommunikation.

MANUEL BOLZ (Universität Hamburg, DE, in Kooperation mit Sabine Wöhlke) beschäftigte sich mit der Kommunikation von Geschlechtszugehörigkeit bei so genannten Trans*-Kindern im klinischen Kontext. Während Diversität bzgl. Religion und Ethnizität mittlerweile im Pflegekontext durchaus ein anerkanntes Problem darstellt, träfe dies für Genderdiversität noch nicht zu. Er untersuchte die Ausbildung und persönlichen Hintergründe von Krankenschwestern, wo er die Problematik verortete. Zwar ging er nicht auf visuelle Repräsentationen ein, plant aber für die Zukunft audiovisuelles Ausbildungsmaterial. Auf die Frage, warum nur weibliches Pflegepersonal befragt wurde, verwies er ebenfalls auf die Fortführung des Projekts, innerhalb derer auch andere bzw. fluide Identitäten und Fragen des Alters Berücksichtigung finden sollen.

Die Künstlerin BARBARA GRAF schloss das Panel mit einem bewegenden autoethnographischen Beitrag ab, innerhalb dessen sie ihre visuellen Darstellungen veränderter Körperwahrnehmungen und Sinnesstörungen im Verlauf ihrer Erkrankung an Multipler Sklerose zeigte. Die Visualisierungen sind nicht symbolischer Natur (z. B. bzgl. Angst oder Hoffnungslosigkeit), sondern verbildlichen Parästhesie-Symptome, zeigen also die eigenen veränderten körperlich-sinnlichen Wahrnehmungen. Entsprechend wurden in der Diskussion Aspekte der nachhaltigen Einbindung in therapeutische Prozesse angesprochen, z. B. inwiefern PatientInnen und TherapeutInnen eine gemeinsame Sprache finden können und ob das Malen/Zeichnen eine transformative Erfahrung oder „Heilung" bewirken könne.

Das letzte Panel des Tages sprach das Thema der Demenz an. HERWIG SWOBODA und RENATE SCHACHNER (Klosterneuburg, AT) stellten den Einsatz von Keramikproduktionen in der geriatrischen ergotherapeutischen Praxis vor. Diese Form der Heilpädagogik stelle keine kurative Praxis dar, ermögliche aber die Verknüpfung sensorischer, affektiver und kognitiver Eindrücke. Der Nutzen liege vor Allem im Potential der Erinnerung, aber auch in Aspekten der Gruppenzugehörigkeit und gegenseitiger Aufmerksamkeit.

In einem weiteren sehr bewegenden Beitrag teilte die Filmemacherin ILEANA GABRIELA SZASZ (Bukarest, RO) ihre persönliche Erfahrung der zunehmenden Demenz ihres Vaters und ihre Strategie, dieser Herausforderung mit der Kamera zu begegnen. Als Resultat präsentierte sie Auszüge ihres ethnographischen Films, der sich insbesondere den zwischenmenschlichen Beziehungen widmet und dem Vater Raum gibt, sich mitzuteilen. So entsteht die Möglichkeit für verschiedene Beteiligte, sich konstruktiv mit einer sich verändernden Lebens- und Gesundheitssituation auseinander zu setzen und auch die sozialen Bezüge von Krankheit zu erörtern.

Der dritte Konferenztag stand ganz im Zeichen der asiatischen, und zunächst der tibetischen Medizin. BARBARA GERKE (Universität Wien, AT) untersuchte die Darstellung von Giften, Ansteckungen und Gegenmitteln in tibetischen Medizin-Thangkas (Rollbilder) aus dem 17. Jahrhundert, die während der therapeutischen Ausbildung die Erinnerung von Texten

unterstützen sollten. Dabei wurde deutlich, dass der Buddhismus nicht nur als Staatsreligion fungierte, sondern auch die Medizin nachhaltig formte: das Wissen um Substanzen und dessen Darstellung basierten auf Mythen, jedoch nicht unbedingt auf Vorstellungen von schwarzer Magie und Hexerei, wie es im christlichen Kontext gang und gäbe war. Stattdessen wurde eher von spirituellen und sozialen Aspekten gesprochen (beispielsweise im Kontext von Nahrung oder Menstruation) und davon, dass gewisse Substanzen gezähmt werden müssen. In der Diskussion wurde angemerkt, dass es hier durchaus Parallelen zur Homöopathie gibt.

Der Mediziner FLORIAN PLOBERGER (Wien, AT) widmete seinen Vortrag der Darstellung von drei verschiedenen Qualitäten des menschlichen Pulses, die in der tibetischen Medizin als konstitutiv für die Gesundheitsverfassung angesehen werden. Diese werden in den Farben blau, gelb, und weiß kommuniziert und mit verschiedenen Energien, aber auch Geschlechtskonnotationen, in Zusammenhang gebracht. Abweichungen von einer bei der Geburt festgestellten Pulsqualität können als Symptom einer Krankheit diagnostiziert werden oder andere Transformationen im Körper indizieren. Dies impliziert insbesondere, dass ein Therapeut die Pulsqualität bei der Geburt kennt, aber auch die Intuition des Arztes spiele eine Rolle.

Im zweiten und letzten Panel des dritten Tages beleuchtete zunächst ISABEL PIRES (Universität Lissabon, PT) sowohl das Phänomen der tatsächlichen Körpermodifikation junger chinesischer Frauen in China und Portugal als auch die Nachbearbeitung von Selfies in sozialen Netzwerken und Medien. Sie konstatierte, dass diese verbreiteten Praktiken sich verändernden kulturellen, körperlichen und geschlechtlichen Idealen Rechnung tragen und es sogar Programme bzw. Apps gebe, die Frauen entsprechend „beraten". Nichtsdestotrotz erkannte sie hier eher eine Form individueller Handlungsmacht anstatt sozialer Kontrolle, was in der anschließenden Diskussion allerdings erheblich hinterfragt wurde.

KATHARINA SABERNIG (Universität für angewandte Kunst Wien, AT) brachte die Zuhörer zurück zur tibetischen Medizin bzw. zu deren anatomischer Terminologie. Ihre Untersuchung historischen und modernen Vokabulars und dessen Veranschaulichung führte sie zu ihrem FWF-Projekt „Gestrickte Körper Materialität", in dem sie innere Organe und deren Gefäßversorgung in konventionellen Farben strickt und dabei auch Farbzuordnungen asiatischer Traditionen berücksichtigt. Auf die Frage, warum sie sich für das Medium des Strickens entschieden habe, erwiderte sie, dass es Menschen erleichtere, menschliche Organe sehen und anfassen zu können. Auch ethische Probleme der Zurschaustellung menschlichen Gewebes entfallen bei Verwendung des textilen Materials. Eine offene Frage blieb, wie bei der Darstellung unsichtbarer Aspekte (z. B. Chi) zu verfahren sei; man war sich darüber einig, dass Unsichtbarkeit durchaus einen Platz in medizinischen Diskursen haben sollte.

Die abschließende Diskussion strich den Wert visueller Präsentation im gesundheitsbezogenen Raum sowohl im edukativen als auch im expressiven und therapeutischen Sinne hervor. Als besondere Bereicherung wurden jene Beiträge empfunden, die sich der Herausforderung stellten, persönliche Krisen mit unterschiedlichen visuellen Medien darzustellen und sozusagen als Betroffene reflektierend normalerweise unsichtbare vulnerable Gesundheitszustände sichtbar werden ließen. Auch wurde die Bedeutung weiterer zukünftiger Forschung zu Sinneswahrnehmungen und Formen der Kommunikation im Heilungskontext und als Kooperationen von beispielsweise MedizinanthropologInnen und TherapeutInnen hervorgehoben. Allerdings wurden auch die Schwierigkeiten angesprochen, solch interdisziplinäre Projekte zu finanzieren und zu realisieren. Hier ergeben sich Herausforderungen für Forschung und Praxis in der Zukunft, derer sich die TeilnehmerInnen in Zukunft verstärkt annehmen wollen. In diesem Kontext sind auch Vorschläge, Ideen und Kritik durch unsere LeserInnen sehr willkommen.

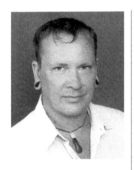

HELMAR KURZ studierte Ethnologie, Religionswissenschaft und Ur- & Frühgeschichte an der Westfälischen Wilhelmsuniversität Münster und promovierte dort 2022 zum Thema „Voices of Good Sense – Diversification of Mental Health and the Aesthetics of Healing in Brazilian Spiritism" im Schnittfeld der Medizin- & Religionsethnologie und Trans/Kulturellen Psychiatrie. Er ist wissenschaftlicher Mitarbeiter am Institut für Ethnologie in Münster und Koordinator des angegliederten internationalen Masterstudiengangs „Visual Anthropology, Media & Documentary Practices" an der WWU Weiterbildung GmbH. Aktuell widmet er sich verstärkt der Bedeutung der Sinne im therapeutischen Kontext und insbesondere darauf bezogener innovativer ethnografischer Methoden innerhalb des Paradigmas der „Ästhetiken des Heilens".

WWU Münster, Institut für Sozial- & Kulturanthropologie
Studtstraße 21, 48149 Münster
helmar.kurz@uni-muenster.de

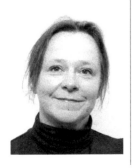

KATHARINA SABERNIG ist Projektleiterin des FWF-Projekts „gestrickte Körper Materialität" (AR-705) an der Universität für angewandte Kunst Wien und studierte Medizin und Kulturanthropologie in Wien. In ihren früheren Projekten beschäftigte sie sich mit anatomischen Illustrationen, visualisierter Medizin und tibetischer medizinischer Terminologie worüber sie zahlreich publizierte. Inspiriert von der Vielfalt der anatomischen Darstellungen und den ethischen Fragen, die mit dieser Kunst verbunden sind, begann sie 2015 mit dem Stricken anatomischer Objekte. In ihrem aktuellen Projekt stellt sie die Topografie der inneren Organe und deren Gefäßversorgung dar, wobei sie sich an den Maßen eines erwachsenen Menschen orientiert.

Universität für angewandte Kunst Wien
Institut für Kunstwissenschaften, Kunstpädagogik und Kunstvermittlung
katharina.sabernig@uni-ak.ac.at

Die Ruhe nach dem Sturm? Medikalisierte Alltage in Zeiten der Covid-19-Pandemie
Bericht zum 19. Treffen des Netzwerks Gesundheit und Kultur in der volkskundlichen Forschung am 7. Juli 2022

ANNA PALM

Am Donnerstag, den 7. Juli 2022 eröffneten SA-BINE WÖHLKE und ANNA PALM, die Sprecherinnen des Netzwerks Gesundheit und Kultur in der volkskundlichen Forschung der Deutsche Gesellschaft für Empirische Kulturwissenschaft (DGEKW), das 19. Arbeitstreffen, das als Onlinetagung stattfand. Nach fast dreijähriger Coronapause kamen, wie auch in den Jahren davor, Wissenschaftler:innen aus verschiedensten Disziplinen zusammen, um über medikale Alltage in Zeiten der Covid-19-Pandemie zu diskutieren. Durch die weltweite Krise haben sich viele Ebenen unseres Alltags verändert, bekannte Ordnungen und Routinen sind aus dem Gleichgewicht geraten. So zeigt sich ein multidimensionales Phänomen, das seither aus vielerlei Richtungen beforscht wird. Neben einer kurzen Einführung, in der die Sprecherinnen für die vielschichtige Thematik sensibilisierten, wurden acht Themen vorgetragen. Die Beiträge verdeutlichen die große Spannbreite der Perspektiven: Akteur:innen im Gesundheitswesen (Pflege, Medizin, Ethik), Wissenschaftler:innen und ihre Familien sowie übergeordnete Fragestellungen nach dem Entstehen neuer Ordnungen und Ebenen der Verantwortung. Das Treffen wurde mit einer Diskussion um die Umbenennung des Netzwerkes und einem Ausblick auf die weitere Planung geschlossen.

Den ersten Vortrag hielt AARON HOCK (Mainz) aus dem Sonderforschungsbereich 1482 Humandifferenzierung der Universität Mainz zum Thema *Pandemische Humandifferenzierung als Alltagsorientierung in Seuchenzeiten*. Nach einer kurzen sozial- und kulturtheoretischen Einführung, in der er das *Doing* bzw. *Undoing differences* erläuterte, zeigte Hock anhand ausgewählter Themenbereiche auf, wie in Zeiten der Covid-19-Pandemie Differenzierungen und Kategorisierungen sichtbar werden. Dabei stellte er die bewusste wie auch unbewusste Grundunterscheidung zwischen Gefährdende und Gefährdete zentral und problematisierte gleichzeitig diese Unterschei-

dung aufgrund der pathogenen Eigenschaften des Virus einerseits sowie aufgrund der höchst differenten Symptomatik der Erkrankung andererseits. So werden durch den gesellschaftlichen Umgang mit der Pandemie auf verschiedenen Ebenen neue Differenzen verhandelt, etwa in Form von Risikogruppen (Alter und/oder Vorerkrankungen) oder über den Immunitätsstatus. Außerdem führt die Aushandlung von Risikofaktoren auch gesellschaftlich zu einer Neubewertung von Räumen (Innen- versus Außenräume), die Orientierung stiftet. Formen der Humandifferenzierung bewegen sich, wie Hock veranschaulichte, aber auch zwischen Orientierung und Stigmatisierung, was sich etwa in der Diskriminierung wie z. B. „Asiat:innen" zeigt. Teilweise verlassen solche Formen der Humandifferenzierung die Welt des Sichtbaren, etwa beim Immunitätsstatus.

Die visuelle Kulturanthropologin SANDRA ECKHARDT (Göttingen) stellte in ihrem Beitrag *Who cares? An Investigation of the Compatibility of Research and Care Work in the Time of COVID-19 and Beyond* drei Forschungsperspektiven eines interdisziplinären Projektes der Universität Göttingen zum Umgang von Wissenschaftler:innen mit der Pandemie vor. Darin wurde die Vereinbarkeit von Wissenschaft und Familienarbeit aus diskurstheoretischer Perspektive anhand einer Analyse öffentlicher Diskurse, aus der Alltagsperspektive mittels qualitativer Sozialforschung und aus einer philosophischen Perspektive vorgestellt. Als Querschnittsthema zeigte sich anschaulich die Frage, wie in Zukunft mit der Vereinbarkeit von Wissenschaft und Care-Arbeit umgegangen werden soll, und zwar weniger als eine reine private Aushandlung, sondern auch als eine gesellschaftliche Debatte. Ziel des Projektes ist es, auch für ein weites Familien- und Wissenschaftsverständnis zu sensibilisieren.

Aus dem Projekt CoronaCare des Instituts für Sozialmedizin und Epidemiologie der Medizinischen Hochschule Brandenburg referierten FRANZISKA KÖNIG und JOSCHUA PAUL zum Thema *Die Stagnation des Sozialen: Bewegung und Bewegt-werden unter den Bedingungen der Covid-19 Pandemie in Deutschland.* Auf Basis von Alltagsdokumentationen, Telefoninterviews (alle drei Monate) und Fragebogendaten untersuchte das interdisziplinäre Forschungsteam Strategien, um soziale Gesundheit in Pandemiezeiten aufrechtzuerhalten. Den analytischen Rahmen dazu bildete das Verständnis, dass soziale Mobilität konstitutiv ist für soziale Bewegung. Dem vorgestellten Ansatz zur Folge machen Menschen verkörperte Erfahrung, wobei zwischen affektiver und physischer Bewegung unterschieden wird: Affektive Erfahrungen sind beispielsweise das Musikhören oder das Berührtsein. Physische Bewegung wird durch Mobilität sichtbar. Anhand von Beispielen aus dem Feld zeigten die Referent:innen auf, wie neue Räume anhand des Bewegtwerdens und des Sich-Bewegens sichtbar werden, sich Unsicherheiten durch fehlende Bewegung manifestieren und Normalität durch die pandemiebedingten Reglementierungen neuverhandelt wurde.

Aus einer medienwissenschaftlichen bzw. medienethnologischen Perspektive stellte MAJA JERRENTRUP (Landshut) die Ergebnisse aus ihrem Forschungsprojekt zu den Veränderungen der Nutzung von Social Media in Pandemiezeiten dar. Dazu unterzog sie Fotos aus 50 Instagram-Profilen verschiedener europäischer Länder einer ethnographischen Inhaltsanalyse. Die Bilder versteht Jerrentrup als Bausteine einer Lebenschronik der Nutzer:innen, die auch etwas über die Strategien der persönlichen Verarbeitung der Krise aussagen können. In der vergleichenden Betrachtung der Quellen zeigt sich ein hoher Anstieg krisenbezogener Motive, etwa durch Fotografien von Personen mit Masken oder begehrter Konsumgüter (wie etwa Klopapier, Mehl, Hefe). Zudem zeichnet sich ein deutlicher Fokus auf das Eigene in Form von Selbst- und Familienportraits oder Bildern von Haustieren ab. Fotografien von kreativen Aktivitäten und Yoga sowie Erinnerungen an vorpandemische Zeiten sieht Jerrentrup als Bausteine einer fragmentierten Identität.

Einer internationalen Perspektive auf Ethik in der Pandemie widmet sich der Beitrag von SABINE WÖHLKE (Hamburg), die das Forschungsprojekt *Medicine & Ethics go viral* des Instituts für Ethik und Geschichte der Medizin der Universität Göttingen und des Instituts für Gesundheitswissenschaften der HAW Hamburg vorstellte. Zentral für das Projekt sind Interviews mit Bioethiker:innen weltweit seit Beginn der Pandemie. Für das Projekt wurden insgesamt 46 Interviews geführt und einer empirisch-ethischen Analyse unterzogen. Im Ländervergleich wird sichtbar, wie nicht nur in Deutschland eine medizinethische Diskussion über die sogenannte Triage bei einer möglichen Verknappung von Intensivpflegeplätzen, sowie Altersrationierung, rechtliche und moralische Pflichten gegenüber bereits versorgten Menschen, Fehlorganisation von Gesundheitsressourcen entbrannt ist. Aber auch die Folgen für vulnerable Gruppen in der Gesellschaft durch Quarantäne und Isolierung werden in Frage gestellt. International treten weitere Themen zu Tage, die andere ethische Bereiche betreffen, wie z. B. die Rationierung des Gesundheitswesens nach rassistischen Gesichtspunkten, gesundheitliche Ungleichheiten und Gesundheitskompetenz zwischen ethnischen, Alters- und Klassengruppen oder die unfreiwillige Überwachung von Mobilität und Kontaktpersonen über Apps und Mobiltelefone und die eingeschränkte Palliativpflege oder familiäre Pflege. Die Interviews werden in einer virtuellen Ausstellung der Öffentlichkeit zugänglich gemacht (www.ethicsgoviral.com). In der Diskussion wird deutlich, welcher Mehrwert das Material für die Erforschung dieser weltweiten Krisensituation einerseits und auch für die Entwicklung von Lehrmaterialien für den medizinischen, pflegerischen und medizinanthropologischen Unterricht andererseits haben kann.

Ein ähnlich gelagertes Projekt stellten EHLER VOSS (Siegen) und MIRKO UHLIG (Mainz) in ihrem Vortrag *Im Auge des Sturms. Autoethnographisches Schreiben während der Pandemie* vor. Gemeinsam initiierten sie mit der *Curare*-Redaktion bereits im März 2020, kurz nach der Erklärung des weltweiten Pandemiezustandes, einen Schreibaufruf: Wissenschaftler:innen waren aufgefordert, über einen längeren Zeitraum autoethnographische Tagebücher im strikten Sinne des Wortes (Malinowski) zu schreiben. Der Aufruf richtete sich an Kultur- und Sozialwissenschaftler:innen und somit an Personen, denen die Methode des autoethnographischen Schreibens vertraut war. So sollten neben Alltagserfahrungen auch kulturelle und medizinische Aspekte im Erleben dieser weltweiten Krisensituation, wie z. B. verschiedene Heiltheorien oder Grußpraktiken, eingefangen werden. Insgesamt wurden 58 Ego-Dokumente, vornehmlich von Kulturanthropolog:innen und Ethnolog:innen aus unterschiedlichen Ländern zusammengetragen und online veröffentlicht. Anhand zweier Beispiele machen Voss und Uhlig deutlich, dass die Texte nicht nur Zeugnisse subjektiver Bewältigung der Krise sind, sondern darüber hinaus in vielen Fällen auch zu einer kulturanthropologischen Interpretation führen. Ethnographische Methode und der Selbstzweck des Tagebuchschreibens verschränkten sich vielfach, so dass hier methodisch herausfordernde Quellen erhoben wurden. Im Nachgang der Erhebung sind bisher zwei Schwerpunkthefte der Zeitschrift *Curare* entstanden, in denen einzelne Schreibende ihre eigenen Texte in einem zeitlichen Rückblick reflektieren. Insgesamt beschreiben die Vortragenden ihr Projekt der Curare Diaries als Experiment, mit dem umfangreiches, heterogenes Material zusammengetragen wurde, das über verschiedene Forschungszugänge erschlossen werden kann.

Ein drittes Schreibprojekt im Rahmen des Netzwerktreffens stellte SABINE WÖHLKE (Hamburg) in ihrem Vortrag *Unsicherheiten Pflegender während der ersten Covid-19-Infektionswelle und ihre Bewältigungsstrategien* vor. Mitte März bis Mitte April 2020 wurden über die Methode des professionellen Pflegetagebuches Daten zu relevanten Ereignissen, Emotionen und Selbstreflexionen der Pflegenden in Bezug zu ihrer Arbeit in der Klinik erhoben. Im Vortrag präsentierte Wöhlke einerseits Ausschnitte aus den gewonnenen Quellen sowie andererseits erste Ergebnisse der Analyse. Aus einer pflegeethischen Perspektive ließen sich verschiedene Ebenen der Verantwortung herausarbeiten, die auch über die berufsspezifische Selbstbestimmung der Pflegenden hinausgehen. Inhaltlich ragen vier Themen heraus: Krisenmanagement, die „unsichtbare Krise", Krisenstimmung und die Bewältigung der Krise. In ihrem Fazit macht Wöhlke deutlich, dass die Perspektive der Pflege im beruflichen wie universitären Alltag stärker einbezogen werden sollte: Über innovative methodische Ansätze, wie das professionelle Tagebuch, bieten Möglichkeiten

der partizipativen Einbindung der pflegerischen Perspektive. Zudem könnten so Interessen von Patienten und Pflegenden besser wahrgenommen werden.

Den letzten Beitrag aus aktuellen Forschungsprojekten lieferte MANUEL BOLZ (Hamburg) mit seinem Vortrag *Pflege und Betreuung von trans*-Kindern und Jugendlichen in klinischen Alltagen während der Pandemie*. Er berichtete aus einem Teilprojekt des Verbundprojektes TRANS*KIDS, das sich dem Thema Geschlechtsidentität/trans* im Arbeitsalltag von Mitarbeitenden, Pflegenden und (medizinischen) Fach- und Verwaltungsangestellten im Gesundheitswesen widmet. Ganz konkret stand die Frage im Mittelpunkt, wie Normen und Werteverständnisse zu stigmatisierendem und diskriminierendem Handeln im Umgang mit trans*-Kindern und -Jugendlichen im Klinikalltag während der Pandemie führen können. Am empirischen Material, leitfadengestützter, semistrukturierter Interviews, zeigte er verschiedene Diskriminierungsdimension auf. Im Kontext der Mitarbeitenden waren dies insbesondere die gestiegene Belastung im Arbeitsalltag, die strengen Zeitregime und die Stellenvakanz, die Versorgungsengpässe, die mangelnde Bezahlung oder der Wegfall von Fort- und Weiterbildungsangeboten. Bei den trans*-Kindern und -Jugendlichen verzögerte sich der Transitionsprozess oder Vernetzungsangebote und trans*-Sprechstunden entfielen.

Im Anschluss an die Vorträge führte ANNA PALM (Aachen) in die Diskussion zur Umbenennung des Netzwerkes ein. Anlässlich der Namensänderung des deutschen Fachverbandes von Deutsche Gesellschaft für Volkskunde e. V. (dgv) in Deutsche Gesellschaft für Empirische Kulturwissenschaft e. V. (DGEKW), die am 22. September 2021 beschlossen wurde, hatten Sabine Wöhlke und Anna Palm im März 2022 Anregungen für eine Namensänderung des Netzwerkes an den E-Mailverteiler gesendet. Auf dieser Basis wurde im Rahmen der Onlinetagung weniger das Für und Wider einer Umbenennung, sondern potenzielle Namensvorschläge sowie die Umwandlung des Netzwerkes in eine Kommission innerhalb der DGEKW diskutiert. Die Veränderung des formalen Status' von einem Netzwerk in eine „klassische" Kommission, wurde von den Anwesenden befürwortet. Dadurch würde im

Kontext der anderen Kommissionen mehr Einheitlichkeit innerhalb der DGEKW erreicht, da diese sich alle ohnehin als Netzwerke zu spezifischen Forschungsfeldern verstehen. Hinsichtlich des Namens entfaltete sich eine kleine Kontroverse über die Weite bzw. Enge der Begriffe Medizinanthropologie und Medikalkulturforschung. Für eine Umbenennung in eine Kommission für Medizinanthropologie (in der DGEKW) sprach die ohnehin seit Jahrzehnten praktizierte Nutzung von Konzepten und Methoden der Ethnologie und Medical Anthropology sowie die Nähe zu den Bezeichnungen anderer internationaler Arbeitskreise aus diesem Themengebiet (z. B. das Netzwerk Medical Anthropology Europe der European Association of Social Anthropology (EASA) oder der US-amerikanischen Society for Medical Anthropology). Die Kritik an der deutschen Bezeichnung Medizinanthropologie fußte auf einer zu stark empfundenen Fokussierung auf den medizinischen Themenkreis und den Begriff der Anthropologie, der ggf. naturwissenschaftlich oder philosophisch verstanden werden könnte. Darin spiegelte sich der Wunsch, die kulturwissenschaftliche Ausrichtung zu betonen, weshalb der zweite Begriff der Medikalkulturforschung von den jeweiligen Bedenkentragenden favorisiert wurde. In der Diskussion einigten sich die Anwesenden jedoch auf die Umbenennung in eine Kommission für Medizinanthropologie in der DGEKW. Der Begriff steht in engem Bezug zum internationalen Begriff Medical Anthropology. Für den Begriff Medizinanthropologie steht die Nähe zu internationalen Arbeitskreisen und die Geläufigkeit des Begriffes. Denn im Gegensatz zur Medizinanthropologie hat sich der Begriff der Medikal-

kulturforschung im Kontext der Benennung des Untersuchungsfeldes im Rahmen der kulturanthropologisch-volkskundlichen Forschung in der Vergangenheit nicht durchgesetzt (WOLFF 2008). Zudem erhoffen sich die Mitglieder des Netzwerkes, durch die neue Bezeichnung als Kommission Medizinanthropologie ein stärkeres Angebot zur Identifikation (TAUSCHEK 2021) zu bieten. Der neue Name würde die bereits seit Jahren gelebte Interdisziplinarität des wissenschaftlichen Austausches über die Disziplingrenzen hinweg stärker nach außen repräsentieren (vgl. VOSS 2018).

Das Netzwerktreffen schloss mit einer kurzen inhaltlichen Abschlussrunde sowie mit einem Bericht der Sprecherinnen über aktuelle Tätigkeiten: So wird in den nächsten Monaten der alte Verteiler in eine DFN-Mailingliste überführt, die Umbenennung mit der DGEKW auf den Weg gebracht sowie eine neue Internetseite der künftigen Kommission erstellt. Für das Jahr 2023 ist bereits eine gemeinsame Tagung mit der Arbeitsgemeinschaft Ethnologie und Medizin (AGEM) vom 8.-9. September 2023 in Hamburg in Planung. Ein Call for Papers findet sich am Ende dieses Hefts.

Literatur

TAUSCHEK, MARKUS 2021. Ein neuer Name setzt ein wichtiges Signal. Zur Umbenennung der Deutschen Gesellschaft für Volkskunde. *Zeitschrift für Volkskunde. Beiträge zur Kulturforschung* 117, 1: 63–73.
VOSS, EHLER 2018. Fröhliche Wissenschaft Medizinanthropologie. *Curare* 41, 1+2: 3–7.
WOLFF, EBERHARD 2008. Patientenbilder. Zur neueren kulturwissenschaftlichen Gesundheitsforschung. *Bricolage* 5: 24–38.

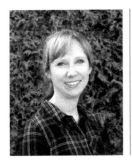 **ANNA PALM** studierte Kulturanthropologie/Volkskunde, Städtebau und Kunstgeschichte. Von 2008 bis 2012 war sie als wissenschaftliche Mitarbeiterin und Mentorin in der Abteilung Kulturanthropologie der Universität Bonn tätig. Seit 2013 arbeitet sie als wissenschaftliche Mitarbeiterin im Zentrum für Hochschuldidaktik und Qualitätsentwicklung in Studium und Lehre der Fachhochschule Aachen (derzeit in Elternzeit). Als externe Doktorandin am Institut für Film-, Theater-, Medien- und Kulturwissenschaft der Universität Mainz hat sie im Oktober 2022 ihre Dissertation verteidigt und ist seit 2012 Sprecherin des Netzwerkes „Gesundheit und Kultur in der volkskundlichen Forschung" der DGEKW.

Zentrum für Hochschuldidaktik und Qualitätsentwicklung der FH Aachen
Goethestr. 3, 52064 Aachen
palm@fh-aachen.de

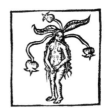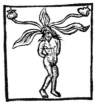

EMILY PIERINI 2020. Jaguars of the Dawn. Spirit Mediumship in the Brazilian Vale do Amanhecer
New York: Berghahn, 278 pp. (20 figures)

EMILY PIERINI is a social anthropologist focusing on the intersection of medicine, religion, spirituality, and healing. She currently works at the anthropology department of Sapienza University of Rome, Italy. This publication is based on her PhD thesis and provides unique insight into mediumship practices in Brazil and beyond. It vividly connects ethnographic accounts with anthropological considerations on well-being and experience. The title of this monography frames the focus of her research: the "Jaguars" are mediums within the community of the "Valley of the Dawn" where the author implemented extensive fieldwork between 2004 and 2018 in Brazil and, due to its translocal networks, in Italy, Great Britain, and Portugal.

She organizes her argument into nine chapters, framed by an introduction, a conclusion, and an appendix that provides a glossary and descriptions of crucial spiritual entities. The chapters each start with narratives from her fieldwork experiences and then follow a specific line of thought embedded in ethnographic data and its anthropological discussion, connecting to the previous and subsequent chapters through the interrelatedness of scopes, concepts, and topics. Thus, PIERINI provides deep insights into her engagement with the field, and the strength of this book is her excellent writing style between vivid narration, clear explanation, and comprehensible discussion that has the reader dive into the author's experiences and perspectives.

She introduces the *Vale do Amanhecer* as a Brazilian movement that since 1959 has combined various spiritual knowledge and practices, e.g., of Afro-Brazilian religions and Spiritism, but also (pre)historical cultures and ideas of astral worlds and space travels. As a central practice, she identifies mediumship as a means of establishing relations with spiritual beings and past-life experiences. She perceives mediumship as a health-related process addressing the body and notions of self. PIERINI decides on a phenomenological approach that links narratives of lived bodily and perceptual experiences to conceptual categories such as embodiment, knowledge,

belief, or feeling, stressing sensory aspects of perception. She focuses on the apprenticeship and cultivation of "multidimensional selves" in therapeutic settings, that is, dynamics regarding the transformation of a sense of self and bodily experience in terms of "permeable bodies" and "extended selves" as particular "ways of knowing" (7). She integrates this idea with her methodology, acknowledging autoethnography and sensory ethnography as ways of "embodied knowledge" (9) that have improved her understanding of her interlocutors' narratives.

Chapter 1 (Ways to Embody the Divine in Brazil) frames the context of her endeavor as a "Brazilian religious meshwork" that identifies as highly diverse and fluid due to the mutual influence of practitioners and their mobility between practices of Afro-Brazilian, Indigenous, Christian, and Spiritist origin and new upcoming movements celebrating the bricolage of notions regarding body and self, communication between humans and non-humans, and health explanatory models. Chapter 2 (The Vale do Amanhecer) narrows down to the history and context of the movement's rise alongside the establishment of the new capital Brasília as a modernist and millenarian project, attracting many new religious movements in the 1960s. The author describes how *Vale do Amanhecer* (VdA) materialized from one person's (Tia Neiva) spiritual experience toward a charitable but hierarchically organized institution and a translocal and international movement that envisions and propagates a new era of spiritual science in nowadays over 700 sites in Brazil and abroad (Europe, US, Latin America, Japan).

Chapter 3 (Jaguars of the Dawn: The Transhistorical Self) introduces the mediums engaging with VdA, who attempt to embody forces of past lives to implement the heritage of all humanity into procedures that aim at nothing less than the healing of humanity as such. It involves ideas on spiritual progress, reincarnation, and karma ever since allegedly 32 000 years ago, spiritual beings from other planets reincarnated on planet Earth and, with time, created the first civilizations, with pyramids and megalithic formations manipulating vital electromagnetic forces. Accordingly, their cosmology is quite global and inclusive but also has a transhistorical character.

Chapter 4 (Spirits in Transition: The Multidimensional Self) draws on spiritual notions of self that relate to these processes of incarnation and disincarnation, forms of exchange with spirit worlds, and related ecologies of fluids and substances, ritual spaces, symbols, and knowledge. Human beings are conceptualized in terms of multiplicity and multidimensionality as consisting of a body, a soul, and a spirit, and thus existing on different (energetical) planes (individually, socially, spiritually) beyond physical aspects:

> Humans are therefore entangled in these fluidic relations with spirits and also with other humans; through thoughts and emotions, they may affect or be affected by other people's energies. This human spirit ecology is what defines 'disobsessive healing' in the Vale do Amanhecer [...] (114).

However, the physical body appears as the center of manipulation and transformation in the context of healing.

Chapter 5 (Disobsessive Healing) introduces to spirit-related aetiologies of health and illness and related therapeutic practices that focus on the attendance of afflicting spirits and their guidance to a hospital on the spiritual plane (also see Kurz 2017: 201). Therapy thus does not reduce to the afflicted human being but extends to his ties with so-called spirit obsessors and past-life encounters that might have caused these entanglements. Aetiologies of illness thus locate between material and spiritual causes, and treatment organizes between spiritual first aid and sustained spiritual treatment alongside mediumship development.

Chapter 6 (Mediumship) elaborates on the notions of mediumship quite different from those of Spiritism, Spiritualism, or Afro-Brazilian religions. According to PIERINI, participants in VdA perceive it as a universal biological and bodily feature that culturally only differs in its practical elaborations. Spirit incorporation is only one of many bodily manifestations of extended sensory experience (see Kurz 2017: 203). It is not per-

ceived as a semi- or unconscious cognitive state of "possession" but as an altered state of bodily perception and "sharing vibrations" (139). Further, mediumistic development means learning "how to become aware of and gain control over one's mediumistic forces and to balance them through their distribution in healing rituals" (140). Those who enter this development do so in several steps of initiation over months and years and have previously passed as patients or their company.

Chapter 7 (Learning Spirit Mediumship: Ways of Knowing) analyzes this process as practical and drawing upon bodily experience. Here, EMILY PIERINI also shares her experiences in an autoethnographic and sensory-ethnographical way, using her body to grasp somatosensory aspects and specific modes of knowing through enskillment, that is, attending to bodily sensations and feelings. She describes mediumship development as increased attention to emotions, feelings, and sensory perceptions and the training of different modalities of expressing energies running through the body by gestural and verbal codes. In doing so, the author stresses aspects previously discussed within Curare as "Aesthetics of Healing" (see KURZ 2017, 2019): healing is perceived as a transformational process of knowing and enskillment beyond conceptional cognition and involves practical, bodily learning.

In a final reflection and discussion, Chapters 8 (Spiritual Routes) and 9 (Therapeutic Trajectories) explore the motivations of participants beyond concepts of "social inclusion" or "religious marketplaces" as individual progress and mobility in terms of the ongoing construction of a sense of self. The author stresses the importance of experiences of sustained transformation and the immediacy of relationships with the divine (or maybe better: the spiritual; note of the reviewer). The notion of healing intertwines with these spiritual routes that may range from experiences of spiritual first aid to mediumship practices that support selves and others complementary to biomedical treatments and with such severe ailments as mental disorders, alcoholism, and drug addiction.

In her conclusion, PIERINI stresses the highly transformative process negotiated along (past) life trajectories on an experience-based, bodily level. She criticizes theoretical discussions that reduce mediumship to pathology, belief, or neurological aspects. Accordingly, she clarifies:

> This analysis is not intended as an exhaustive explanatory paradigm of what is a complex process of spiritual healing. I rather intended to focus upon embodied knowledge to illuminate specific dynamics that emerged from my interlocutors' narratives upon the therapeutic uses of mediumistic development; and I did so in the light of my approach to the processes of initiatory learning as a multilayered experience – which is embod-

ied, intuitive, performative, conceptual and intersubjective, articulating particular notions of the body and the self. (224)

HELMAR KURZ, Münster

References

KURZ, HELMAR 2017. Diversification of Mental Health: Brazilian Kardecist Psychiatry and the Aesthetics of Healing. *Curare* 40, 3: 195–206.
KURZ, HELMAR (ed) 2019. The Aesthetics of Healing: Working with the Senses in Therapeutic Spaces. *Curare* 42 (3+4).

JENNY HUBERMANN 2021. Transhumanism. From Ancestors to Avatars
Cambridge: University Press, 292 pp.

JENNY HUBERMAN is Associate Professor of (Cultural) Anthropology at the University of Missouri, Kansas City, USA. She investigates practices, values, and visions among US-American Transhumanists who imagine a future where science and technology will enable humanity to overcome alleged biological, mental, and physical limitations for the sake of creating a somewhat posthuman species and society. To start with, she shares her observation that experiences of loss, mourning, and memorialization are changing and that our contemporary digital age might promote mind cloning technologies as a new step in human evolution, an idea that she imagines as rather alien and horrifying:

> Did I really want to live in a world where my great, great grandmother's digital avatar would join me for Thanksgiving dinner? Or my grandparents would be cared for by "cyberconscious" robots? Or my mindclone digital offspring called "bemans" would "stage civil rights movements" to ensure they "win the same status that flesh-and-blood humans enjoy" [...]? [...] This is completely crazy! (1)

However, HUBERMAN sovereignly approaches the field as an anthropologist who enters new terrains and throughout this rich monography, she repeatedly refers to classical ethnographies to frame her investigation of this contemporary cultural phenomenon that appears to sustainedly

shape human future – not to say that it is already reengineering the human species to usher in a posthuman future:

> [...] I came to realize that transhumanists are interested in using science and technology to reconfigure conceptions of the person, the body, kinship, cosmology, the social and political order, and the physical environments in which our future descendants will dwell. (2)

She, therefore, pursues to answer the question of "[h]ow does the transhumanist understanding of the world; of human nature, the person, kinship, cosmology, the good life, and so on, *compare and contrast* with the way human beings, living in other times and places, have conceived of such things" (3)? HUBERMAN understands transhumanism as a sociocultural movement to enhance capabilities and to overcome limitations toward a "humanity+". She aims to investigate

> [h]ow are new forms of technology reconfiguring human life in the twenty-first century? How are technologists assuming an ever-greater role in shaping the future of our species? And more specifically, how does 'the technological imagination' [...] become a powerful force in the making of social lives and futures? (5f)

Other topics are radical life extension, colonialization of space, achieving immortality through mind cloning, developing robots with a full range of human cognitive abilities, using technology to achieve eternal bliss and new forms of body augmentation, acquiring powerful capabilities, and counteracting the deficiencies of aging, illness, and death. These ideas have had an impact on TV series and movies, but also on the industrial development of self-driving cars and military technologies to augment the bodily and cognitive abilities of soldiers. Accordingly, transhumanist projects are already real in remaking the social, material, and imaginative worlds we live in. Body- or biohackers use chips to enhance their sensory capacities and promote a defective understanding of human nature and the substituting possibilities of neurobiology, computer sciences, and artificial intelligence. HUBERMAN observes that the transhumanist movement mainly consists of highly educated, predominantly white, male elites, who share libertarian outlooks in the US with a robust commitment to capitalism, whereas, e. g., in pre-1989 Russia, divergent political perspectives would have shaped techno enthusiasm alongside alleged future social(ist) approaches. Thus, one question to state is on how visions of transhuman technologies would serve the existential needs of populations or, once again, the economical greed of a few (as we may also observe in contemporary biomedical technologies).

HUBERMAN's declared aim of the book is to provide 1) an anthropological exploration of transhumanism as a contemporary socio-cultural movement and its visions, values, practices, and projects and 2) to introduce students to new fields of anthropology by using classical anthropological comparative methods. She discusses the diverging and converging frames of religion and science in the context of "late modernity" (12), where new religious movements advance technoscientific ideologies *and* science-based cosmological visions. Accordingly, she does not perceive transhumanism as antithetical to religion but instead discovers blurred lines with secular interests of economic and cosmological significance: a new form of capitalism that is allegedly dedicated to species salvation and new ideas of social organization. Methodologically, she implements approaches in digital ethnography to explore discussion forums, blogs, websites, and other related media that discuss the use of science and technology to improve human life. Complementary, she

reports of public events where she has participated in and conducted (narrative) interviews.

Apart from her introduction and conclusion, HUBERMAN structures this monography in seven chapters. Chapter 1 (*Is Transhumanism a Revitalization Movement?*) juxtaposes the religious and social natures of transhumanism by integrating ANTHONY WALLACE's (1956) work on revitalization movements. HUBERMAN considers explanatory models of responses to social stress and attempts of creating a more satisfying culture where available technologies would eliminate the distress of aging and enhance human intellectual, physical and psychological capacities. This perspective predicates a profound dissatisfaction with the current human condition and the biological chains that keep human beings from actualizing their fullest potential. According to the author, this mind frame developed throughout the cultural distortions of the Cold War where apocalyptic dreads would nourish divergent responses from evangelicalism to transhumanism in the USA.

Chapter 2 (*Ancestors and Avatars: Immortality Transformed*) focuses on immortality initiatives of mind cloning and compares them to practices of dealing with human existential dilemmas such as reproduction and survival. By referring to MEYER FORTES (1987), HUBERMAN compares practices of "making avatars" to those of "making ancestors". Accordingly,

> [a]ncesterhood has thus been a desirable means of constructing the afterlife because it reaffirms relationships and practices that are widely recognized as maintaining sociality and vitality among the living (55).

Making avatars, in terms of mind uploading and/or a transfer of consciousness, involves robotic bodies, body repletes, or holographs to construct the afterlife but even more reaffirms core values of a late capitalist society that envisions a posthuman age instead of a continuity of humanity's wellbeing.

In Chapter 3 (*Happily Ever After: Transhumanism and the Hedonistic Imperative*), HUBERMAN elaborates on a related aspect of a "good life" and "happiness" as being framed by specific social contexts and values of what transhumanists perceive as worthy. In reminiscence of RUTH BEN-

EDICT (1934) and MICHAEL JACKSON (2011), she addresses the topic of how socio-cultural rather than biological needs shape individual desires and accordingly elaborates on how the hedonistic imperative shapes visions and attempts of living "happily ever after" by promoting rationality, scientific progress, evolutionary biology, and materialism. I cannot help myself to think about the cyborg species of the *Borg* within the *Star Trek* universe here. Instead of addressing class inequality, racism, sexism, bigotry, nationalism, and all other forms of structural violence producing human suffering, the solution for human affliction is sought in synchronization, rationalization, consumption of perfecting drugs, and other forms of biochemical engineering.

Subsequently, Chapter 4 (*The Social Skin, the Antisocial Skin, and the Pursuit of Morphological Freedom*) critically explores the pursuit of "morphological freedom", that is, the individual's right to modify their body according to one's desires. With reference to TERENCE TURNER (1980), it reflects on "social skins" as bodies being betwixt and between a unique self and shared meanings and values they reproduce. To make things more complicated and even have the reviewer reflect on how much he already might be a transhumanist himself, HUBERMAN introduces TURNER's student ROSENBLATT (1997) who investigates so-called "modern primitives" and their forms of body modification (tattoos, piercings, scarifications, etc.) as a means of communicating estrangement from modern society, expressing resistance, and performing an "authentic self" in terms of a symbolically represented nonconformity to standards of Western capitalist society (even though I want to add that many related practices have been commodified in recent years and nowadays it almost seems to be a symbol of enhanced nonconformity *not* to apply to these practices). Interestingly, HUBERMAN even in this context of an alleged asexual optimization of human existence detects gender discourse in terms of "technomasculinity": "We're not a bunch of hippy, dippy bongo players with dreadlocks hanging out and having fun, we actually make shit, we get shit done!" (110)

These stereotypes guide me to Chapter 5 (*Decoding the Self*) where HUBERMAN deconstructs conceptions of self within this informatic, quantified, and databased cross-fertilization between neurosciences, computer sciences, and AI in comparison to HALLOWELL's (1955) notions of personhood and self-awareness beyond other-than-human scopes. How do we conceptualize the self and how do conceptions influence behaviors and practices? Is the human body the seat of consciousness and self? HUBERMAN does not explicitly address but implicitly touches on the reviewer's concerns: what about the senses, feelings, affections, emotions, and aesthetics? More than any other chapter of this book, this one warns of forgetting who we *are* for the sake of some alleged scientific progress that reduces to cognitive knowledge and neglects the impact of sensory experience. Hollywood movies (e. g., *Matrix*, *The Lawnmower Man*, etc.) have illustrated the dangers of such approaches, nonetheless "the market" urges us to increasingly apply to them, with certain computer apps that we may trust more than our gut feelings and interhuman relationships.

Chapter 6 (*Rethinking Kinship Systems*) thus addresses questions that the reviewer deems scary: does kinship in the posthuman future include digital offspring, robotic kin, or new forms of biological reproduction? What is family? How do we relate to others? Who or what are relatives and/or others? And what about gender and sex markers? Can we leave them behind for the sake of a posthuman kinship that develops from biological to vitological where reproduction is not dependent on married male-female couples anymore but on "rationalized" reproductive acts that do not lead to autonomous offspring with their own identity but rather generate copies of the genitors' selves and/or asexual duplications? Suddenly, it does not appear so futuristic anymore, once related linguistic terms already shape our concerns of "political correctness". On the other hand, it also represents the contemporary sex industry with increasing resources of AI sex robots that imitate empathy and reproduction technologies promoting designer babies and selective reproduction. The reviewer thinks that it is not too much mental gymnastics to imagine what comes next, and has already been before: how to deal with alleged biological "abnormalities"? HUBERMAN addresses all these questions and remains quite objective on these troubling issues. She communicates her discomfort but steps back to analyze both: the transhumanist discourse *and* her personal bias.

In chapter 7 (*From Original Affluence to Posthuman Abundance*), HUBERMAN summarizes values, visions, tensions, and reflections on what a posthuman future might entail for cultural anthropology. Wondering how transhumanists would imagine the future in economic terms, the author imagines divergent approaches among postscarcity, radical abundance, and related socio-political impacts that may or may not direct toward "affluence without abundance" (183). She reflects on SAHLIN's (1972) elaborations on hunter-gatherer-societies and questions regarding the democracy of property, productivity, division of labor, environment, and technological innovation (185ff), outlining that affluence such as poverty results from social structures and relations (187). Accordingly, we must question how health and wealth interrelate, especially when transhumanists pretend to be technophilanthropists while at the same time performing as profit-oriented social entrepreneurs (202ff). How does consumption negotiate individual, socio-political, and economical needs (205f)? Does the promise of technology apply to forces of equality, that is, does it serve social needs or individual satisfaction, or are both interrelated (215)? Does technological progress involve human progress in terms of democratic socialism (216) or does it simply regress into radical capitalism where the gap between rich and poor increases, and the former invest in their immortality by vampyrizing the latter?

In her conclusion (*Back to the Future: Reflections on a Discipline and a Movement*) HUBERMAN does not provide answers to these questions but stresses the fact that transhumanists as a "radical other" challenge future anthropological research to do so (217) by "listening to ancestor anthropologists and their approaches" (222) for the sake of understanding the posthuman future envisioned by transhumanists where technology plays a paramount role in the constitution and organization of both the species and society (224):

> The technological imagination, therefore, does more than provide an entertaining diversion from the "reality" of life. It inspires people, in this case very powerful ones, to create realities in accordance with particular visions of the world as it "could or should be". (235)

To the reviewer, it also involves to further critically exploring biomedical hegemony as an alleged means to improve human wellbeing, including discourse on the obligation to live (on), forced vaccination, reproduction technologies, and, last but not least, plastic surgery for the sake of responding to social expectations of maximum performance.

HELMAR KURZ, Münster

References

BENEDICT, RUTH 2005 (orig. 1934). *Patterns of Culture*. Boston: Mifflin.

FORTES, MEYER 1987. *Religion, Morality and the Person: Essays on Tallensi Religion*. Cambridge: University Press.

HALLOWELL, ALFRED I. 1955. *Culture & Experience*. New York: Shocken.

JACKSON, MICHAEL 2011. *Life Within Limits: Well-Being in a World of Want*. Durham: Duke University Press.

ROSENBLATT, DANIEL 1997. The Anti-Social Skin: Structure, Resistance, and "Modern Primitive" Adornment in the United States. *Cultural Anthropology* 12, 3: 237–334.

SAHLINS, MARSHALL 1972. *Stone Age Economics*. New York: de Gruyter.

TURNER, TERRANCE 2017[1980]. The Social Skin. Reprint. *Hau* 2, 2: 486–504.

WALLACE, ANTHONY 1956. Revitalization Movements. *American Anthropologist* 58, 2: 264–281.

Juli Zeh 2021. Über Menschen
München: Luchterhand, 412 S.

Vor dreizehn Jahren schrieb Juli Zeh mit *Corpus Delicti* einen mittlerweile zur Schullektüre gewordenen dystopischen Roman, der eine gesellschaftliche Situation beschreibt, in der der Umgang mit Krankheit und Tod dem sehr nahekommt, was gegenwärtig viele in der Protestszene gegen die Pandemie-Politik am Horizont des Corona-Diskurses und entsprechender Maßnahmen aufkommen sehen und häufig auf den Begriff der Corona-Diktatur bringen. Dementsprechend meldete sich auch Juli Zeh bald nach der formalen Feststellung einer „epidemischen Lage von nationaler Tragweite" im März 2020 öffentlich zu Wort und machte wie viele andere die Erfahrung, dass Kritik am Regierungskurs und einer ihn stützenden Medienberichterstattung schnell mit der Gefahr verbunden war, unabhängig von Inhalt und Person mit einem Verweis auf ebenjene kritisierte Medienberichterstattung die intellektuelle und moralische Zurechnungsfähigkeit abgesprochen zu bekommen.

Statt weiterer öffentlicher Interventionen in den tagesaktuellen Medien hat sie ein Jahr später mit *Über Menschen* eine Art Corona-Roman veröffentlicht, der die mit der Ausrufung eines Ausnahmezustands entstandene und anhaltende Konfusion thematisiert, die diejenigen in der Protestszene ereilt hat, deren Welt durch die in ihrem sich politisch links verortenden Milieu dominierende gleichgültige bis affirmative Haltung gegenüber einem als autoritär und übergriffig empfundenen Staat in schwindelerregendem Tempo in Stücke zerfallen ist und nach einem ebenso schmerzhaften wie lustvollen und nicht selten einem Erweckungserlebnis gleichkommenden Prozess der Neuzusammensetzung sozialer Beziehungen und politischer Kategorien und Allianzen in völlig neuer Gestalt vor ihnen liegt: Plötzlich scheinen ihnen die einzigen vernünftigen Stimmen zu den sogenannten Corona-Maßnahmen und den damit verbundenen Grundrechtseinschränkungen vor allem aus der Springer-Presse und von AfD-Abgeordneten zu kommen, obwohl man es doch gewohnt war, die autoritären Charaktere hauptsächlich im Boulevard und bei den Rechten zu erkennen und ihnen zu unterstellen, die Bezugnahme auf Demokratie, Meinungsfreiheit und den Schutz der „kleinen Leute" nur als Tarnung zu nutzen, um dahinter ihre eigene chauvinistische Agenda im Interesse eines autoritären Staats und großer Konzerne durchzusetzen; und plötzlich erscheinen ihnen weniger ihre neuen befremdlichen Bettgenossen von Propaganda manipuliert als die sich für gegen Propaganda immun haltende und dadurch für sie an Naivität kaum zu überbietende Vertrauensgemeinschaft der Linken.

Juli Zehs Roman spielt in der Anfangszeit dieser durch die ungewohnte Vermischung und partielle Einigkeit rechter und linker Akteure entstandene Verwirrung während des ersten sogenannten Lockdowns in Deutschland und ist aus der Sicht von Dora geschrieben. Sie ist Mitte dreißig, westdeutsch, stammt aus einer Arztfamilie und hat, wie rückblickend erzählt, bis vor kurzem standesgemäß in Berlin-Kreuzberg zusammen mit ihrem Freund Robert gelebt, der sich zunehmend dem Kampf gegen den Klimawandel verschreibt und zum Teil unnötig überzogen als fanatischer Greta-Groupie karikiert wird, der mit dem Flugzeug ihren Vortragsreisen für mehr Klimaschutz folgt. Robert bringt Dora dazu, ihren Job in einer herkömmlichen Werbeagentur aufzugeben und zu einer Agentur für nachhaltige Produkte zu wechseln – vermutlich als Symbol gedacht für eine sich links verstehende Politik, die nicht mehr die Systemfrage stellt, sondern sich damit zufriedengibt, der kapitalistischen Logik einen grünen Anstrich zu geben, ohne sich der eigenen epistemischen Notlage bewusst zu sein.

In dieser Firma fühlt sich Dora eigentlich ganz wohl und entwirft dort gerade in selbstironischer Appropriation des diffamierend gemeinten Begriffs eine Kampagne für die Jeans-Marke „Gutmensch" des Berliner Start-ups FAIRkleidung, verspürt aber dennoch ein vages Unbehagen an der Moderne, das sich unter anderem mit einem unruhigen Kribbeln und stechenden Schmerzen durch spezifische körperliche Symptome andeutet. Das liegt zum einen an dem ständig drohenden Burnout durch das Multitasking und die Projekte-Kreislauf-Falle der modernen Lebens- und Arbeitswelt, die es ihr unmöglich machen, einfach nur aus dem Fenster zu sehen, zum anderen aber auch an der Selbstgerechtigkeit ihres klimaaktiven Freundes, der zunehmend unversöhnlich, rechthaberisch und aggressiv versucht, anderen Menschen seine Vorstellung vom guten vernünftigen Leben aufzudrängen und dabei die Paradoxien seines eigenen Handelns nicht erkennt.

Deswegen hatte sich Dora schon in der Zeit vor Corona auf die unbestimmte Suche nach einer Ausstiegsoption gemacht und dabei heimlich ein verwildertes Haus im ländlichen Brandenburg gekauft. Doch erst als ihr Freund seine Identität als apokalyptischer Klimareiter mit der des Zeugen Coronas vervollkommnet und in dieser Doppelrolle wie berauscht mit Kassandrarufen in seinen Online-Kolumnen mediale Erfolge als Corona-Experte feiert – eine Art des Krisengewinns, für die man reale Vorbilder nicht lange suchen muss –, verweigert sich Dora endgültig dem von ihrem Freund eingeforderten Treuschwur auf die Apokalypse. Sie ist befremdet von Roberts Gefühl der Überlegenheit des eigenen Lebensstils, welches sich dennoch von den verachteten Lebensentwürfen provozieren lässt, ebenso wie von seiner undifferenzierten Gleichsetzung ihrer Kritik an sich auf unumstößliche Wahrheiten berufende Autoritäten mit Donald Trumps Rede von alternativen Fakten.

Roberts Versuch, Dora aus Infektionsschutzgründen das Gassigehen mit ihrem Hund zu untersagen, bringt das Fass zum Überlaufen. Sie verlässt ihn und mit ihm Berlin und zieht auf ihr neu erworbenes Flurstück in dem bereits aus ZEHS Roman *Unterleuten* bekannten Dorf Bracken – in einer Gegend, in der die Alternative zum Diesel nicht, wie in den Städten, teurer Nahverkehr, sondern gar kein Nahverkehr ist und zu den unsolidarisch und sozial unausgeglichen erscheinenden Klimakonzepten von „denen da oben" die vermeintliche Alternative für Deutschland. Corona und entsprechende Schutzmaßnahmen spielen hier auf dem dünnbesiedelten Land außer in Witzen keine Rolle, aber nicht wie bei Doras Vater aus einem großbürgerlich-elitären Selbstverständnis heraus, demzufolge die Regeln für das niederere Volk für ihn natürlich nicht gelten, sondern weil es sich bei Corona aus Sicht der Dorfbewohner*innen ohnehin nur um eine weitere „Volksverarschung" handelt.

In Bracken, wo der Roman beginnt und endet, trifft Dora auf das, was die Moderne seit ihren Anfängen als ihr Gegenteil konstruiert und erfolglos und zum Teil mit gegenteiligem Effekt auszuschließen versucht hat: das Primitive, Animalische, Rückständige, Lächerliche, Hedonistische und Brutale, als das auch die aktuellen Proteste gegen die Corona-Maßnahmen immer wieder kategorisiert werden, und das gleich nach ihrer Ankunft in Gestalt des Dorf-Nazis Gote auf dem Nachbargrundstück zum Vorschein kommt. Als Echo der großen Trennung von Moderne und Nicht-Moderne treffen mit Dora in Bracken gleich mehrere gewöhnlich asymmetrisch konstruierte Dichotomien aufeinander: Stadt-Land, Westen-Osten, Oberschicht-Unterschicht. Dabei scheinen sich ihr zunächst alle Klischees des Primitiven zu bestätigen. So widmet sich ihr Nachbar vor allem seiner Rauschkultur, ist ungehobelt im Umgang mit ihr und anderen, brutal zu ihrem Hund, isst das Fleisch ohne Salat, wohnt allein in einem einfachen Bauwagen, lässt sein Haus und seine Tochter verwahrlosen, hat nach der Wende mit seinem Vater Geflüchtetenunterkünfte angezündet und singt das Horst-Wessel-Lied zusammen mit seinen Freunden, mit denen er bis vor kurzem noch wegen eines Messerangriffs auf ein linkes Städterpaar im Gefängnis saß.

Doch je länger sich Dora in Bracken aufhält, desto mehr wandelt sich das Verhältnis zu ihrer Umgebung. Das Fremde wird für sie langsam zu einem gesuchten und gefundenen Spiegel, in dem sich der Blick auf das Eigene und damit auch das Fremde verkehrt und das Fremde die Erfüllung der eigenen Sehnsüchte verspricht. So verkehrt sich etwa das verbreitete Klischee der Eintönigkeit des Dorfes und der Vielfältigkeit der Stadt in sein Gegenteil, wenn sich Bracken als eine überraschend heterogene Existenzgemeinschaft mit hoher Widerspruchstoleranz und einem ungezwungen fürsorglichen Miteinander entpuppt, in der scheinbar Unvereinbares mehr oder weniger friedlich koexistiert oder sich vermählt. Konfrontation und Kooperation mit dem fremden Anderen wird im Dorf durch ihre Unvermeidlichkeit erst ermöglicht, während eine Annäherung an das fremde Andere in der Stadt durch das Beziehungsideal des Gleichklangs, das ihren Ausdruck in den Finetuning-Optionen der Dating-Apps findet, möglichst vermieden wird.

Dementsprechend kommt Dora in Bracken auch nicht um eine Annäherung an den für sie lächerlichen Übermenschen in feingerippten Unterhemden aus dem Nachbarhaus herum und langsam gesellen sich zu der von ihr empfundenen Unsicherheit, Angst und Abscheu irritierende Gefühle der Freundschaft bis hin zur Anziehung, wenn hinter der barbarischen Oberfläche Gotes nach und nach die Figuren des verletzlichen Kindes, liebevollen Vaters, naturverbundenen Tierfreunds, fürsorglichen Nachbarns, selbstvergessenen Künstlers und spirituell überlegenen – sozusagen rechtsesoterischen – primitiven Philosophen hervortreten, die anders als Dora und ebenso wie die immer wieder auftauchende und eine Romantisierung des Animalischen aufrufende in sich ruhende Katze in der Lage sind, im Jetzt zu leben, die Welt so wie sie ist und das Denken sein zu lassen und Dora dabei zu der Erkenntnis verhelfen, dass in Bracken wie auf der ganzen Welt die Mutter aller Probleme die Ansicht ist, etwas Besseres zu sein als die anderen.

Um das Buch zu einem Corona-Roman zu machen, dürfen natürlich auch Reflexionen über Krankheit und Tod nicht fehlen, wobei Corona jedoch nie als konkrete Infektion, Erkrankung oder gar Todesursache auftritt, sondern nur als Diskurs, was der Wahrnehmung vieler Maßnahmenkritiker*innen entspricht, die auf Teufel komm raus darauf bestehen, dass Covid-19 mit einer gewöhnlichen Grippe gleichzusetzen und die Außergewöhnlichkeit einer pandemischen Situation ein reines Medienereignis ist, hinter dem sich ein verabsolutiertes Gesundheitsideal und eine Tendenz zur Negation des Todes abzeichnet, welche ähnlich wie in *Corpus Delicti* beschrieben, nur in einen Totalitarismus führen können, und die dabei nicht selten das Kunststück vollbringen, gleichzeitig von einer Harmlosigkeit des Virus und einem Ursprung im Labor auszugehen. Und dieser in *Über Menschen* auftauchende Diskurs über den abwesenden Erreger ist vor allem ein auch aus der Protestszene bekannter polemisch-kritischer, der sich entweder auf die Momente des Vergessens der pandemischen Lage oder auf die wahrgenommenen Irrationalitäten der Schutzmaßnahmen und menschlichen Verhaltensweisen konzentriert, wenn etwa Dora über die Uneinigkeit der Experten reflektiert; sie sich wundert, dass Leute, die

unbesorgt mit 140 km/h auf der Bundesstraße fahren, gleichzeitig Angst vor Krankheiten haben können; ihr Ex-Freund Robert als jemand erscheint, der Biertrinker vor dem Spätverkauf für gemeingefährliche Volksverräter hält; Doras Vater das Anspruchsdenken für die wahre Pandemie hält und über diejenigen den Kopf schüttelt, die wochenlang Corona-Tagebücher schreiben, Corona-Regeln befolgen, Corona-Talkshows gucken, Corona-Gespräche führen und in den Kommentarspalten Lockerungsbefürwortern den Tod wünschen und davon plötzlich nichts mehr wissen wollen, sobald der Pfingsturlaub beginnt; oder andersherum, wenn Dora sich über die Outlaws im Anpassungsmodus lustig macht, als sich die Nazi-Freunde Gotes an die staatlich verordneten Abstandsregeln halten.

Konkret kommen Krankheit und Tod am Ende aber doch noch ins Spiel, als das Leben des völkischen Raumforderers durch eine innere Raumforderung bedroht wird und der menschliche Neonazi nach vollendetem Kunstwerk seine Souveränität über den Tod durch einen Selbstmord beweist. Und dann ist es Doras Vater, der ihre eigenen irrationalen Hoffnungen auf eine Auslöschung des Todes mit dem im Corona-Diskurs tabuisierten Satz begegnet, „er wäre sowieso bald gestorben", um etwas später hinterherzuschicken, „wer den Tod akzeptiert, kann damit leben".

Die sich aus einer unfreiwilligen Allianz entwickelnde uneingestandene Liebesgeschichte zwischen der linksliberalen westdeutschen Stadtbewohnerin aus besserem Hause und dem unterschichtigen rechtsradikalen Dorfbewohner aus Ostdeutschland findet ihren Abschluss mit Gotes Beerdigung, mit der Dora, nachdem sie von ihrer Werbeagentur mit herzlichen Grüßen entlassen worden ist, als seine vorgebliche Witwe vollends zu einem Teil der Dorfgemeinschaft wird; durch den Tod wendet sie sich dem Leben zu, der beginnende Frühling deutet mit singenden Vögeln und klappernden Störchen die ewige Wiederkunft an und der letzte Satz den berühmten Blick – schwer von Geduld, Heiterkeit und gegenseitigem Verzeihen – den ein unwillkürliches Einverständnis zuweilen auszutauschen gestattet mit einer Katze.

Mit ihrem Roman über die edlen Wilden aus Brandenburg hat JULI ZEH den Nerv eines großen Teils der politisch rechts wie links ausgerichteten und die Querfront-Geschichte häufig positiv rezipierenden deutschen Protestszene gegen die Corona-Maßnahmen getroffen, der vor dem Hintergrund der eigenen Wahrnehmung, dass ein die Verhältnismäßigkeit der Maßnahmen infragestellender Querschnitt der Bevölkerung für die Erinnerung daran, dass Grundrechte keine Leckerli, sondern Abwehrrechte gegen den Staat sind, als staatsfeindlich und nach dem Prinzip pars pro toto von der Mehrheit als rechtsextrem oder rechtsesoterisch diffamiert wird, den Schluss zieht, die Kategorien links und rechts hätten für die politische Diskussion heutzutage keine Bedeutung mehr und seien zugunsten der Kategorie einer gemeinsamen großen und aus welchen Gründen auch immer harmonisch visionierten Menscheitsfamilie zu beerdigen.

Außer Acht gelassen wird dabei jedoch oft, dass die Verwischung des Unterschieds zwischen rechts und links das traditionelle Geschäft der Rechten ist, die in diesem Fall die antikapitalistischen und egalitären Impulse vieler zum Teil neu politisierter und von den Linken alleingelassener und dadurch in die Arme der Rechten getriebener Maßnahmenkritiker*innen zu ihren Gunsten zu nutzen wissen, indem sie ihnen oft unbemerkt den Stachel ziehen und ins Gegenteil verkehren. Somit steht zu befürchten, dass JULI ZEHS romanhafter Gegenwartskommentar eher zur weiteren Verwirrung als zur dringend nötigen Aufklärung der Situation beiträgt.

EHLER VOSS, Bremen

ZUSAMMENFASSUNGEN
ABSTRACTS
RÉSUMÉS

Zusammenfassungen der Beiträge der *Curare* 45 (2022) 2

Schwerpunkt „Lebensanfänge und -enden. Ethnographische Erkundungen und methodologische Reflexionen"

HERAUSGEGEBEN VON JULIA REHSMANN & VERONIKA SIEGL

JULIA REHSMANN & VERONIKA SIEGL Lebensanfänge und -enden als Brennglas für die ethnographische Forschung. Einleitung zum Special Issue S. 7–16, verfasst auf Englisch

MARCOS FREIRE DE ANDRADE NEVES Afterlife Reverberations. Praktiken der Namensgebung in der ethnografischen Forschung zur Sterbehilfe S. 17–27, verfasst auf Englisch

Können ethische Entscheidungen die Menschen überleben, die sie getroffen haben? Gestützt auf ethnografische Forschung zur Sterbehilfe, wirft dieser Artikel einen kritischen Blick auf die Auswirkungen von Praktiken der Namensgebung nach dem Tod, insbesondere die Verwendung von Anonymisierung und Pseudonymen. Akteure, die um die gesellschaftliche und politische Anerkennung von Sterbehilfe kämpfen, organisieren eine spezifische Namenspolitik, die ethischen Anforderungen innerhalb der der akademischen Sozial- und Kulturanthropologie widerspricht, die Anonymität zum Schutzes von Forschungsteilnehmer*innen zu wahren. Diese Dissonanz schafft eine Situation, in der eines der wichtigsten Schutzinstrumente der Sozial- und Kulturanthropologie Gefahr läuft, die politischen Kämpfe derjenigen Menschen zu konterkarieren, die es zu schützen versucht. Vor diesem Hintergrund argumentiert dieser Beitrag, dass die empirische Erforschung von Tod und Sterben eine zusätzliche Sensibilität für Namensgebung erfordert. Daher schlage ich den Begriff der *afterlife reverberations* vor, der die Affekte und Erwartungen beschreibt, die sich nach dem Tod von Forschungsteilnehmer*innen aus im Leben getroffenen Forschungsentscheidungen heraus entwickeln.

Schlagwörter Anonymität – Sterbehilfe – Forschungsethik – Pseudonym – Namensgebung

MIRA MENZFELD Liminale Asymmetrien. Übergangsdynamiken in Beziehungen zu Sterbenden – ein Verstehensansatz S. 28–38, verfasst auf Englisch

Der vorliegende Artikel bietet eine Option für ein ethnologisch informiertes Verständnis von onto-hierarchischen Besonderheiten an, die die Beziehungen zwischen nichtsterbenden Personen, z. B. Forscher:innen, und sterbenden Gesprächspartner:innen charakterisieren und mitgestalten können. Der Text stützt sich auf Feldforschungen mit ansprechbaren Personen, die 1) an einer unheilbaren Krankheit litten, 2) über ihre unheilbare Prognose informiert wurden und 3) diese Art von Diagnose als verlässliche Information über ihr eigenes Sterben einstuften. Ich beziehe mich auf klassische Turner'sche Ideen von Schwellen- und Übergangsdynamiken, um einen wichtigen Faktor zu verstehen, der Forschungsbeziehungen mit bewusst Sterbenden durchdringt und manchmal schwierige Situationen während der Feldforschung hervorrufen kann: Diesen Faktor nenne ich liminale Asymmetrie. Liminale Asymmetrien zeichnen sich durch mindestens drei Dimensionen aus: Erstens die Tatsache, dass sich Sterbende in einem Zwischenzustand befinden und dementsprechend den Wunsch nach liminaler Begleitung und Führung im Sterben haben können (nicht-todkranke Menschen sind nicht in der Lage die Rolle eines liminalen Führers oder Begleiters volladäquat auszufüllen, weil sie sich nicht in einem vergleichbaren Zwischenzustand befanden oder befinden). Zweitens eine entscheidende Erfahrungshierarchie: Sterbende besitzen einen privilegierten Zugang zu einer Seinsweise, die Nicht-Sterbende noch nicht erfahren haben. Drittens eine weitere existenzielle Hierarchie: Sterbende – nachdem sie eine unheilbare Diagnose als verlässliche Aussage über ihre Gegenwart und Zukunft anerkannt haben – sehen sich in der Regel in einem weniger privilegierten Zustand des Seins, der Handlungsfähigkeit und der Lebendigkeit als Nicht-Sterbende. Wenn wir liminale Asymmetrien als prägend für Sterbeerfahrungen anerkennen, erhalten wir ein zusätzliches Instrument zum Verständnis von Forschungssituationen, in denen liminale Asymmetrien direkt oder indirekt thematisiert werden. Der Artikel stellt zwei exemplarische Feldforschungsszenarien vor, um zu veranschaulichen, welche Arten von Situationen als Verhandlungsarenen der (Un-)Möglichkeiten von liminaler Begleitung und liminaler Führung sowie von fähigkeitsbezogenen Hierarchien identifiziert werden können.

Schlagwörter Sterben – teilnehmende Beobachtung – Liminalität – liminale Asymmetrie – terminale Erkrankung

Molly Fitzpatrick Unbehagliche Fürsorge *(care)*. Herausforderungen des „Zusammen-seins" *(being with)* als Doula-Ethnografin   S. 39–51, verfasst auf Englisch

Anthropolog:innen, die empirisch zu Lebensanfängen und – enden forschen, verspüren oftmals das Bedürfnis eine aktive Rolle in der Fürsorge *(care)* ihrer Forschungsteilnehmer:innen einzunehmen. Der vorliegende Beitrag bietet eine Reflektion über meinen Versuch während meiner ethnografischen Feldforschung zu Geburtspraktiken in zwei Hebammenkliniken auf Bali, Indonesien, Fürsorge *(care)* als Doula, einer nicht-medizinischen Geburtshelferin, zu leisten. Die Rolle der Doula-Ethnografin bedeutete eine Verschiebung meiner Rolle im Geburtssetting, weg von stiller Beobachtung und „Da-sein" *(being there)*, hin zu einem „Zusammen-sein" *(being with)* mit Gebärenden. Wie ich in diesem Beitrag darlege, basiert dieser Modus des „Zusammen-seins" auf Ideen des Bezeugens und Miterlebens *(witnessing)*, sowie einer offenen Haltung gegenüber Interaktionen und Momenten. Anhand meiner Forschungserfahrungen zeige ich auf, dass diese Art der Fürsorge *(care)* auch mit Unbehagen und komplexen ethischen Überlegungen verbunden war. In meinem Artikel argumentiere ich für die Notwendigkeit, dieses Unbehagen ernst zu nehmen und zu reflektieren und zeige auf, wie mich die affektiven Aushandlungen meiner Fürsorge *(care)* gegenüber gebärenden Frauen zu wesentlichen ethnografischen Einsichten geführt hat.

Schlagwörter Geburt – Ethnografie – Doula – Fürsorge/*Care* – Affekt

Forschungsartikel

Jürgen W. Dollmann Eine interdisziplinäre Betrachtung von „Ganzheitlichkeit" in Komplementär- und Alternativmedizin   S. 55–68, verfasst auf Deutsch

Komplementäre und alternative Medizinverfahren werden häufig mit dem Begriff der „Ganzheitlichkeit" unter Einbindung von Körper, Geist und Seele angeboten und rezipiert. Dieses Konzept, das im vorliegenden Beitrag im Zentrum steht, wird oft nicht nur als Abgrenzung zur Schulmedizin herangezogen, sondern häufig auch mit spirituellen Aspekten verbunden. Ein Grund dafür kann darin gesehen werden, dass viele komplementär- und alternativmedizinische Verfahren wie beispielsweise Ayurveda und Traditionelle Chinesische Medizin aus dem südbzw. ostasiatischen Bereich stammen und zum Teil aus religiösen bzw. philosophischen Traditionen abgeleitet werden. Der Autor, selbst Internist und Kulturwissenschaftler, führt historische und kulturwissenschaftliche Aspekte der „Ganzheitlichkeit" mit kognitions- und neurowissenschaftlichen Erkenntnissen zusammen. Eigene Feldforschungsergebnisse im Bereich des Ayurveda werden exemplarisch angeführt. Zur Integration dieser interdisziplinären Betrachtung dienen sogenannte Embodiment- oder Verkörperungstheorien, mit welchen die sinnliche Erfahrung von Akteurinnen und Akteuren im Untersuchungsfeld analysiert werden können. Der Ganzheitsbegriff kann aus dieser Perspektive als anschlussfähig an die spirituellen Aspekte der komplementär- und alternativmedizinischen Verfahren gesehen werden. Im Zentrum dieser Arbeit steht die Frage, wie und warum von Seiten der Patientinnen und Patienten eine „Ganzheit" erfahren und sinnlich erlebt werden kann. Die Frage nach der *Wirksamkeit* dieser Medizinverfahren wird nicht berührt. Die Positionalität des Verfassers ist explizit interdisziplinär und mehrperspektivisch, wodurch angestrebt werden soll, blinde Flecken der verschiedenen Medizinverfahren aufzudecken. Die hier vorgenommene Methodentriangulation kann zu Ambiguitäten führen, die jedoch als Diskussionsanregung zwischen kultur- und naturwissenschaftlichen Perspektiven verstanden werden sollen. In einem Resümee werden Anregungen gegeben, die helfen könnten, dem Ausgrenzungsdiskurs der unterschiedlichen Heilsysteme entgegenzuwirken. Das Ziel ist die weitere Förderung einer Integrativen Medizin.

Schlagwörter Komplementär- und Alternativmedizin – Evidenzbasierte Medizin – Ganzheitsmedizin – Integrative Medizin – Embodiment – Spiritualität

Article Abstracts of *Curare* 45 (2022) 2

Thematic focus "Beginnings and Ends of Life. Ethnographic Explorations and Methodological Reflections"

EDITED BY JULIA REHSMANN & VERONIKA SIEGL

JULIA REHSMANN & VERONIKA SIEGL The Beginnings and Ends of Life as a Magnifying Glass for Ethnographic Research. Introduction to the Special Issue   p. 7–16, written in English

MARCOS FREIRE DE ANDRADE NEVES Afterlife Reverberations: Practices of Un/naming in Ethnographic Research on Assisted Suicide   p. 17–27, written in English

Can ethical choices outlive the people who make them? In order to explore this question, this article draws on ethnographic research on transnational assisted suicide to question afterlife implications of practices of un/naming, particularly the use of anonymisation and pseudonyms. Assisted suicide is organised around a specific politics of naming that animates its fight for social and political recognition but which contradicts anthropology's once long-standing disposition towards anonymity as a form of protecting research participants. This dissonance creates a situation where one of anthropology's main tools of protection risks jeopardising the political struggles and fight for recognition of the same people it seeks to protect. Against this background, this reflection argues that empirically researching death and dying requires an additional sensitivity to un/naming practices. Thus, I propose the notion of afterlife reverberations, that is, the affects and expectations that ripple in the aftermath of a research participant's death from their research choices made in life.

Keywords anonymity – assisted suicide – research ethics – pseudonym – un/naming

MIRA MENZFELD Liminal asymmetries. Making sense of transition dynamics in relations with dying persons   p. 28–38, written in English

The article presents one option for an anthropologically informed understanding of onto-hierarchical particularities that can characterize and shape relationships between non-dying persons (e. g. researchers) and dying interlocutors. The article draws on research with responsive and conscious persons who 1) suffer from a terminal illness, 2) have been informed about their terminal prognosis, and 3) regard their diagnosis as reliable information about their own dying. The classic Turnerian ideas of *threshold* and *transition dynamics* are applied to make sense of *liminal asymmetry* as an important factor that permeates research relations with consciously dying persons and can sometimes create challenging situations during fieldwork. Liminal asymmetries are characterized by at least three dimensions. First, as dying persons are in a 'betwixt-and-between' state, they often desire liminal companionship and guidance when dying. (Persons who are not terminally ill are inherently incapable of adequately fulfilling the role of liminal guide or companion because they are not in a state of betwixt-and-between.) Second, the experience of hierarchy is crucial, as the dying have privileged access to a mode of being that the non-dying have not yet entered. Third, as another existential hierarchy, dying persons –

having accepted a terminal diagnosis as a reliable statement about their presence and future – usually consider their state of being, agency, and vitality to be less privileged than that of non-dying persons. By acknowledging liminal asymmetries as formative for experiences of dying, we gain an additional tool for understanding research situations in which liminal asymmetries are directly or indirectly thematized. The article describes two exemplary fieldwork scenarios to illustrate the types of situation identified as arenas for negotiating the (im)possibilities of liminal companionship and liminal guidance, as well as capability-related hierarchies.

Keywords Dying – participant observation – liminality – liminal asymmetry – terminal illness

MOLLY FITZPATRICK Uncomfortable Care. Feeling through Ways of 'Being With' as a Doula-Ethnographer   p. 39–51, written in English

When doing research at the beginning and end of life, ethnographers often feel the urge to engage in the care of the people they are studying. In this paper, I reflect on my attempts to provide care as a volunteer doula, a non-medical birth support person, while conducting ethnographic fieldwork on childbirth in two midwifery clinics in Bali, Indonesia. Becoming a doula-ethnographer meant going beyond silent observation – what might be called 'being there' – to 'be with' women in labour. In this article, I explore this mode of being with, and show how it centres on witnessing, letting things happen, and not going in with an agenda. As my experiences show, caring in the mode of being with was also often uncomfortable and riddled with complex ethical considerations. In this paper, I stay with and reflect on this discomfort to show how the affective negotiations of my attempts to care for women in labour led me to crucial ethnographic insights.

Keywords childbirth – ethnography – doula – care – affect

Research Articles

JÜRGEN W. DOLLMANN An Interdisciplinary Analysis of "Holism" in Complementary and Alternative Medicine   p. 55–68, written in German

Treatments in complementary and alternative medicine are regularly articulated and adopted via the concept of "holism", involving body, mind, and soul. This concept, which is at the heart of this contribution, is not only brought up in distinction to conventional medicine, but often connected to spiritual ideas. One reason for this can be seen in the fact that many treatments in complementary and alternative medicine such as Ayurveda and Traditional Chinese Medicine descend from South Asian and East Asian contexts and are – in part – derived from religious or philosophical traditions. The author, who is both, a specialist in internal medicine as well as a scholar of culture, brings together historical and culture-theoretical aspects of "holism" with insights from cognitive science and neuroscience. The author's research findings from the context of Ayurveda are discussed paradigmatically. To integrate this interdisciplinary analysis, this paper makes use of so-called theories of embodiment, which allow to analyze the sensorial experience of social actors in the given field of research. From this perspective, the notion of "holism" can be regarded as compatible with spiritual aspects of treatments from complementary and alternative medicine. At the heart of this contribution lies the inquiry as to how and why patients can sensually experience "holism". The question pertaining to the efficacy of such medical treatments is not touched upon. The positionality of the author is explicitly interdisciplinary and multi-perspectival which intends to reveal the blind spots of various medical treatments. The methodical triangulation presented here can lead to ambiguities which should be seen as a stimulation for further discussion between culture-theoretical and (natural)science-oriented perspectives. In sum, several suggestions are offered to counteract the exclusionary discourse of various healing systems. The goal is to further promote integrative medicine.

Keywords complementary and alternative medicine – evidence-based medicine – holistic medicine – integrative medicine – embodiment – spirituality

Résumés des articles de *Curare* 45 (2022) 2

Dossier thématique « Débuts et fins de vie. Explorations ethnographiques et réflexions méthodologiques »
SOUS LA DIRECTION DE JULIA REHSMANN & VERONIKA SIEGL

Julia Rehsmann & Veronika Siegl Les débuts et les fins de vie. Des révélateurs pour la recherche ethnographique. Introduction au numéro spécial p. 7–16, rédigé en anglais

Marcos Freire de Andrade Neves Afterlife Reverberations. Dé-nommer comme pratique dans la recherche ethnographique sur le suicide assisté p. 17–27, rédigé en anglais

Les choix éthiques peuvent-ils survivre aux personnes qui les font? Afin d'explorer cette question, cet article s'appuie sur la recherche ethnographique sur le suicide assisté transnational pour questionner les implications après la mort des pratiques de dé/nommer, en particulier l'utilisation de l'anonymisation et des pseudonymes. L'assistance au suicide s'organise autour d'une politique spécifique de la dénomination qui anime son combat pour la reconnaissance sociale et politique mais qui contredit la disposition ancienne de l'anthropologie à l'anonymat comme forme de protection des participants à la recherche. Cette dissonance crée une situation où l'un des principaux outils de protection de l'anthropologie risque de mettre en péril les luttes politiques et de lutter pour la reconnaissance du même peuple qu'il cherche à protéger. Dans ce contexte, cette réflexion soutient que la recherche empirique sur la mort et le mourir nécessite une sensibilité supplémentaire aux pratiques de dé/nommage. Ainsi, je propose la notion de réverbérations après la mort, c'est-à-dire les affects et les attentes qui se répercutent au lendemain de la mort d'un participant à la recherche à partir de ses choix de recherche faits dans la vie.

Mots clés anonymat – Le suicide assisté – éthique de la recherche – pseudonyme – dé/nommer.

Mira Menzfeld Asymétries liminales. Donner un sens à la dynamique de transition dans les relations avec les personnes mourantes p. 28–38, rédigé en anglais

L'article présente une approche pour une compréhension anthropologiquement informée des particularités onto-hiérarchiques qui peuvent caractériser et façonner les relations entre les personnes non mourantes, par exemple les chercheurs, et les interlocuteurs mourants. Le texte s'appuie sur des recherches menées auprès de personnes réactives et conscientes qui 1) souffrent de maladies en phase terminale, 2) ont été informées de leur pronostic final et 3) considèrent ce type de diagnostic comme une information fiable sur leur propre mort. Les idées turneriennes classiques de dynamique de seuil et de transition sont appliquées pour donner un sens à un facteur important qui imprègne les relations de recherche avec les personnes consciemment mourantes et qui peut parfois créer des situations difficiles pendant le travail de terrain : l'asymétrie liminale. Les asymétries liminales sont caractérisées par au moins trois dimensions : Premièrement, le fait que les personnes mourantes se trouvent dans un état intermédiaire et, par conséquent, ont souvent le désir d'être accompagnées et guidées dans leur mort (alors que les personnes qui ne sont pas en phase terminale sont intrinsèquement incapables de remplir adéquatement le rôle de guide ou de compagnon liminal, car elles ne se trouvent pas dans un état intermédiaire). Deuxièmement, une hiérarchie d'expérience cruciale : les mourants possèdent un accès privilégié à une modalité d'être auquel les non-mourants n'ont pas encore accédé. Troisièmement, une autre hiérarchie existentielle : les mourants – après avoir reconnu un diagnostic de phase terminale comme une déclaration fiable sur leur présence et leur avenir – se considèrent généralement dans un état moins privilégié d'être, d'action et de vivacité, par rapport aux non-mourants. En reconnaissant que les asymétries liminales façonnent les expériences de mort, nous obtenons un outil supplémentaire pour comprendre les situations de recherche dans lesquelles les asymétries liminales sont indirectement ou explicitement thématisées. L'article fournit deux scénarios de travail de terrain exemplaires pour illustrer les types de situations identifiées comme des arènes de négociation des (im)possibilités d'accompagnement liminal et d'orientation liminale, ainsi que les hiérarchies liées aux capacités.

Mots clés mourir – observation participante – liminalité – asymétrie liminale – maladie terminale

MOLLY FITZPATRICK Inconfortable soin *(care)*. Ressentir à travers diverses façons « d'être avec » *(being with)* en tant que doula-ethnographe p. 39–51, rédigé en anglais

Lorsqu'ils/elles font des recherches sur le début et la fin de vie, les ethnographes ressentent souvent le besoin *(care)* de s'impliquer directement auprès des personnes qu'ils/elles étudient. Dans cet article, je présente mes réflexions sur mes tentatives de prendre soin *(care)* de mes interlocutrices en tant que doula bénévole, une assistante non médicale d'aide à la naissance, tout en menant un travail ethnographique de terrain sur l'accouchement dans deux cliniques de sage-femmes à Bali, en Indonésie. La posture de doula-ethnographe supposait d'aller au-delà de l'observation silencieuse – ce que l'on pourrait appeler « être là » *(being there)* – pour « être avec » *(being with)* les femmes parturientes. Dans cet article, j'explore cette façon d'être avec, et je montre comment elle est centrée sur le fait d'être témoin *(witnessing)*, de laisser les choses se produire, et de se défaire de nos idées préconçues. Comme le montrent mes expériences, s'impliquer dans le soin *(care)* sur le mode de l'accompagnement est souvent inconfortable et miné de considérations éthiques complexes. Dans cet article, j'explore cet inconfort et montre comment les négociations affectives liées à mes tentatives de m'impliquer auprès des femmes parturientes m'ont conduite à des questions ethnographiques fondamentales.

Mots clés accouchement – ethnographie – doula – soins – affect

Articles de recherche

JÜRGEN W. DOLLMANN Etude interdisciplinaire sur la globalité de l'être humain dans les médecines complémentaires et alternatives p. 55–68, rédigé en allemande

Des procédures de médecine complémentaire et alternative sont souvent proposées avec la notion de globalité de l'être humain qui implique le corps, l'esprit et l'âme, et de même prescrites. Ce concept qui est au centre de l'article présent, n'est pas seulement allégué pour établir les limites par rapport à la médecine officielle, mais il est aussi fréquemment lié à des aspects spirituels. Une raison peut en être que beaucoup de thérapies des médecines complémentaires et alternatives, comme par exemple Ayurveda, la Médecine Tradictionnelle Chinoise, sont originaires de l'Asie du sud ou de l'est et qu'elles découlent de traditions religieuses et philosophiques. L'auteur, lui-même spécialiste de médecine interne et scientifique culturel, met en relation les aspects historiques et culturels de la globalité de l'être humain avec les connaissances cognitives et neurologiques. Les résultats de ses recherches scientifiques sur le terrain, dans le domaine de l'Ayurveda sont donnés en exemples. Des théories d'embodiment ou cognition incarnée, avec lesquelles les expériences sensorielles des acteurs dans le champs d'étude peuvent être analysées, servent d'intégration à cette étude interdisciplinaire. La notion de globalité peut être considérée, dans cette perspective, comme lien avec les aspects spirituels des procédures de médecine complémentaire et alternative. Au centre de cette étude, la question est de savoir, comment et pourquoi les patients et les patientes peuvent faire l'expérience d'une globalité et la vivre sensoriellement. La question de l'efficacité de ces procédures de médecine n'est pas évoquée. La positionnalité de l'auteur est explicitement interdisciplinaire et avec plusieurs perspectives, c'est pourquoi il est nécessaire de découvrir les taches aveugles des différentes procédures de médecine. La triangulation méthodique effectuée ici peut mener à des ambiguités qui cependant doivent être comprises comme une incitation à faire une discussion entre les perspectives sozio-culturelles et scientifiques. Dans un résumé, des incitations sont données qui pourraient aider à éviter un débat d'exclusion des différents systèmes curatifs. Le but est la promotion d'une médecine intégrative.

Mots clés médecine complémentaire et alternative – médecine basée sur les faits probants – médecine holistique – médecine intégrative – cognition incarnée – spiritualité

ANTHROPOS 117.2022

Articles

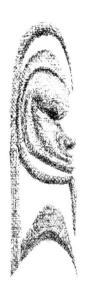

James W. Turner: Controversies Revisited. A Defense of the Concept of Religion

Alberto Saviello: Natürlich Katholisch?! Die Präsentation außereuropäischer Kulturen und nichtchristlicher Religionen im historischen Missionsmuseum der Societas Verbi Divini in Steyl

Hebe A. González y Silvia Hirsch: Abordaje etnolingüístico y etnográfico de las prácticas y conocimientos en torno a la salud reproductiva en comunidades tapiete de la Argentina

Félix Ntep Massing: La sorcellerie et la creation des entreprises en Afrique. Eléments de compréhension théoretique de leur association

Matthias Egeler, and Carola Lentz: Things that Place Names Do. Comparative Perspectives from West Africa and Iceland

Geger Riyanto: Assimilating Stranger, Exemplifying Value. The Realization of Ideal Cultural Representation and Upland-Lowland Relationship in North Seram, Eastern Indonesia

Tian Guang: The Development of Business Anthropology in China

Konstantinos Zorbas: Shamanism and Cultural Evidence of Intangible Violence in Tyva, Siberia

Book reviews by:

J. J. Rivera Andía, J. N. Baumann, M. Beck, I. Blumi, J. Boomgaarden, C. Clados, P. Destrée, T. Dunn, M. Eckholt, J. Estermann, M. F. Fontefrancesco, A. Harms, J. K. Jacka, H. Kroesbergen, O. Gächter, C. J. Gardner, H. Grauer, S. Grodż, A. Gunsenheimer, N. Hellmann, P. Henke, W. Matthews, L. K. Moko, M. F. Morton, J. Pauli, J. Philipps, M. C. Rossi, M. Schindlbeck, B. E. Schmidt, V. Špirková, S. Steindl-Kopf, K. Riede, B. Riese, J. Riese, S. Ruderer, M. L. Tjoa-Bonatz, H. F. Vermeulen, E. P. Wieringa, H. Zinser

ANTHROPOS is published twice a year totalling more than 700 pages.

Individual subscription 2 issues per annum, incl. Online € 98.00 (single-site access); Students € 39.00 (singel-site access); Firms/Institutions € 158.00, multiple use, unrestricted number of online users (either access data or IP address)

Subscription orders should be sent to: Nomos Verlagsgesellschaft mbH, D-76530 Baden-Baden, Germany, E-Mail: orders@nomos.de

Manuscripts and books to be reviewed be addressed to: Anthropos Redaktion, Arnold-Janssen-Str. 20, D-53757 Sankt Augustin, Germany; Fax: 02241-237491; E-Mail: editorial@anthropos.eu

ACADEMIA 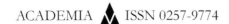 ISSN 0257-9774

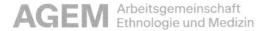
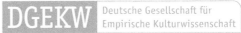

CALL FOR PAPERS

Krisen, Körper, Kompetenzen. Methoden und Potentiale medizinanthropologischen Forschens

35. Jahrestagung der Arbeitsgemeinschaft Ethnologie und Medizin (AGEM)
in Kooperation mit dem 20. Arbeitstreffen der Kommission Medizinanthropologie
der Deutschen Gesellschaft für Empirische Kulturwissenschaft (DGEKW)
vom 8.–9. September 2023 im Warburg-Haus in Hamburg

Krisen und die Rede von Krisen haben Konjunktur. Neben Umwelt, Versorgungs, und Finanzkrise haben nicht zuletzt die Verbreitung von SARS-CoV-2 und die damit verbundenen erheblichen sozialen, politischen, gesundheitlichen und wirtschaftlichen Folgen vielen vor Augen geführt, wie fragil Gesellschaften und gesellschaftlicher Zusammenhalt sind. Krisen- und Liminalitätserfahrungen stellen soziale Ordnungen in ihren alltäglichen Selbstverständlichkeiten in Frage und sind im sozialen Wandel bspw. an Übergängen des Lebensverlaufes wie Geburt, Schuleintritt, Pubertät, Berufswahl, Partnerschaft, Kinder, Ruhestand oder drohender Tod selbst alltäglich. Als persönliche Krisen können sie das Leben erschüttern, z. B. durch die Diagnose einer unheilbaren oder chronischen Krankheit oder durch den Verlust eines nahestehenden Menschen und Risse in der eigenen Biographie verursachen, die, neben unvorhergesehenen Ereignissen, durch intersektionale soziale Marginalisierungen, bspw. im Kontext von Disabilities, verstärkt werden. In der gegenwärtigen Situation spitzt sich die Frage nach den in Krisen eingebundenen Körpern weiter zu.

Mit dieser Tagung richten wir den Fokus auf die medizinanthropologische Erforschung der alltäglichen Erfahrungen und körperlichen Dimensionen von Krisen. Wir fragen nach den Verkörperungen permanenter Krisenerfahrungen und Modifikationen der sinnlichen Wahrnehmung und des Erlebens, die in ihren Folgen selbst im Gesundheitssystem relevant werden, ebenso wie nach deren Bewertungen im Spannungsfeld von Degeneration und Resilienz als verlorene oder gewonnene Kompetenzen. Gleichzeitig fragen wir nach den Potentialen medizinanthropologischen Forschens und laden dazu ein, methodologische Fragen gegenstandsbezogen zu diskutieren. Zentral für diese Diskussion sind unter anderem kollaborative und partizipative Forschungsansätze, die die konventionelle Dichotomie der Forschenden und der zu Erforschenden hinterfragen. Die medizinanthropologische Forschung zeigt, wie Gesundheitsideen und praktiken soziale Ungleichheit nicht nur zum Ausdruck bringen, sondern auch perpetuieren und verstärken können. Mögliche weitere Fragen sind, welche Herausforderungen sich bei der Erforschung körperlicher Erfahrung und sinnlicher Wahrnehmungen für das ethnographische Schreiben ergeben, welche methodologischen Neuerungen, die vor allem durch die pandemische Ausnahmesituation entstanden sind, das qualitative Forschungsspektrum der Medizinanthropologie erweitern und welche neuen Wege zur Reflexion digitaler Forschungsmethoden sich eröffnet haben.

Keynote: Prof. Dr. Hella von Unger (LMU München)

Die Tagung ist interdisziplinär ausgerichtet und wendet sich an Wissenschaftler*innen aus Ethnologie, Europäischer Ethnologie/Kulturanthropologie, Medizinanthropologie, Soziologie, Geschichte, Geschlechterforschung, Medizin, Religions- und Medienwissenschaft sowie angrenzenden Disziplinen. Dabei möchten wir explizit auch Nachwuchswissenschaftler*innen einladen, sich am interdisziplinären Austausch zu beteiligen. Die Tagungssprache wird Deutsch sein.

Interessierte werden gebeten, ein Abstract ihres Vortragsthemas (500 Wörter) zusammen mit einer Kurzbiographie bis zum 31. Mai 2023 an folgende Adresse zu senden: krisen_koerper_kompetenzen@agem.de

AIMS & SCOPE

Die Zeitschrift *Curare* bietet seit 1978 ein internationales und interdisziplinäres Forum für die wissenschaftliche Auseinandersetzung mit medizinanthropologischen Themen, die sämtliche Aspekte von Gesundheit, Krankheit, Medizin und Heilung in Vergangenheit und Gegenwart in allen Teilen der Welt umschließt.

Alle wissenschaftlichen Forschungsartikel werden nach einer ersten Durchsicht durch das Redaktionsteam einer externen Begutachtung im Doppelblindverfahren unterzogen. Alle anderen Beiträge werden von der Redaktion intern begutachtet. Neben Forschungsartikeln werden auch Tagungsberichte und Buchbesprechungen veröffentlicht. Die Rubrik Forum bietet darüber hinaus Raum für essayistische Beiträge, Interviews und ethnographische Vignetten.

Curare publiziert Beiträge auf Englisch und als einzige Zeitschrift für Medizinanthropologie auch auf Deutsch. Sie unterstützt die Publikation von Schwerpunktheften durch Gastherausgeberschaften.

Bei Interesse an der Veröffentlichung eines Beitrages oder der Übernahme einer Gastherausgeberschaft freuen wir uns über eine Email an: curare@agem.de Nähere Informationen zu den Bedingungen von Artikeleinreichungen und Gastherausgeberschaften finden Sie unter: agem.de/curare

Since 1978, *Curare. Journal of Medical Anthropology,* has provided an international and interdisciplinary forum for the scientific discussion of topics in medical anthropology, understood as encompassing all aspects of health, disease, medicine and healing, past and present, in different parts of the world.

After a first internal review by the editorial team, all research articles are subject to a rigorous, double-blind external review procedure. All other submitted manuscripts are internally reviewed by the editorial team. In addition to research articles, the journal publishes conference reports and book reviews. Furthermore, the journal's forum section offers space for essayistic contributions, interviews and ethnographic vignettes.

Curare is unique among medical anthropology journals in that it publishes articles in English and German. *Curare* also supports the publication of guest-edited special issues.

If you are interested in submitting an article or a special issue proposal, please send an email to: curare@agem.de For further information on manuscript submission and guest editorships, please see: agem.de/curare